Guide to becoming a
PHYSICIAN
SECOND EDITION

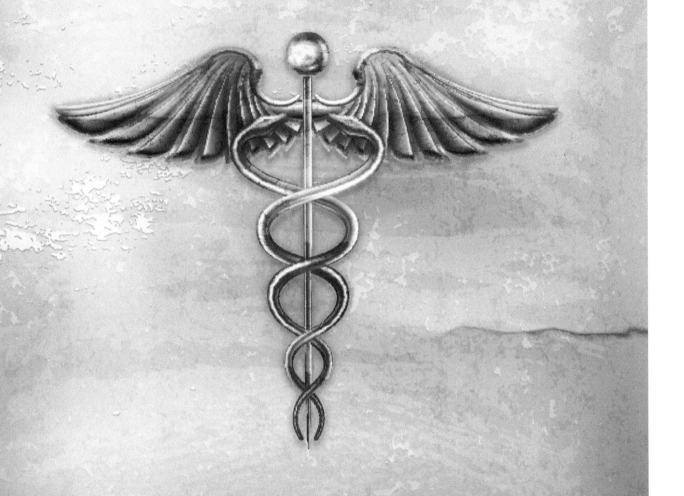

RICHARD SANKER ▪ LEILA E. HARRISON
BOBBIE ANN ADAIR WHITE

Kendall Hunt
publishing company

Kendall Hunt
publishing company

www.kendallhunt.com
Send all inquiries to:
4050 Westmark Drive
Dubuque, IA 52004-1840

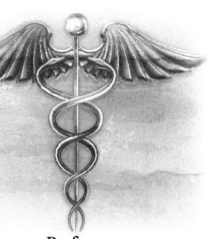

Contents

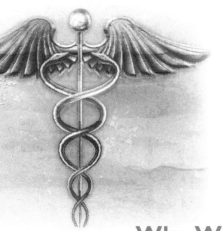

Preface

Why We Wrote This Book

Richard Sanker

I have spent over fourteen years advising and working with premedical students. Their aspirations for their future careers and personal goals have always inspired me to support their educational efforts. There are many students that start their undergraduate careers in the premedical program, but only a fraction of the students are able to advance into medical school. Many struggle with the premedical curriculum or find it challenging to engage with the health professions through shadowing or health related volunteer work. It is puzzling why such talented and intelligent students are so easily frustrated by the process to become a physician.

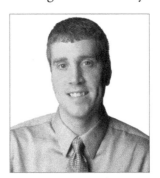

Courtesy Richard Sanker

After many conversations with a variety of undergraduates and personally witnessing so many students either fail in their professional pursuits, or on the other end, make the efforts to persevere through extreme personal and educational struggles, it became evident that students who simply knew and understood why they wanted to become a medical doctor were always more successful in their efforts. To clarify, the premedical students who realized and embraced their personal values and goals would always make their education and professional extracurricular activities their top priority. Regardless of the challenges—be it a difficult semester of courses, personal issues with family or friends, or illness—these students would always put forth their best efforts and end each semester with the grades and accomplishments that would allow their future applications to medical school stand out.

On the other hand, students who lack the professional and personal awareness always seem to struggle with the coursework or never found the time to actively participate in the premedical extracurricular activities. They lacked the motivation necessary to prepare for the premedical classes or to study for the MCAT examination. They seemed to doubt their abilities and were always uncertain about what they needed to do to be competitive for medical school. For a few students, once they realized their professional interests and understood their aspirations for a medical career, they would be more successful in their premedical coursework. More importantly, some students would discover that a career in medicine was not for them and then found success in other professional and academic areas.

Consequently, I wanted to develop and write a book that would help students to recognize and know both the emerging and current responsibilities of the medical doctor so that they can better understand their professional ambitions. A career in medicine is certainly wonderful and exciting, but it requires great effort and sacrifice from the individuals pursing it. Please, take the time and effort to discover what is involved in a medical career and know what the process is to become a physician. Hopefully, this knowledge will inspire your ambitions and give you the motivation to persevere and thrive in your future undergraduate career and medical training.

Leila E. Harrison

When Rich first approached me to co-author this book with him, I was immediately excited. Every day I encounter people who find the admissions process and overall pathway to becoming a physician daunting and perhaps impossible. Others have misconceptions about what a career in medicine entails. This book will serve as a useful, practical guide for people deciding on medicine. I know this guide will reach far more people than I speak to in my office or on the phone, therefore, I'm excited to contribute to this project.

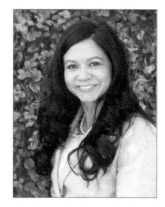

Courtesy Leila E. Harrison

I view my career as having the honor to witness (and sometimes have a role in) the journey people go through in pursuing their passion to serve others through medicine. This book is another great opportunity to contribute to that process. In my many advising sessions, I have encountered those who are still at the superficial stage and do not know where to begin. Others may have started down the road but something may have happened (such as earning a low grade) that has led them to believe their dream is no longer possible. Finally, there are those who have done everything necessary and require little guidance. There are important steps along the way that will help anyone determine whether this is the pathway they want to pursue.

I have found that students who have taken the time to ask "why medicine" and develop a more in-depth response are more likely to find deeper fulfillment in their career. My hope is the response is underlined with the realities of the profession, supported through experiences that expose them to the career allowing them to be more adaptive to the ups and downs and long hours required. Thus, my hope is that this book will help individuals explore the profession from a broader perspective as a whole while understanding each step along the way.

Being a doctor is not a right; it is a privilege. It is a pathway that requires strong work ethic, determination, adaptability, and sacrifice. These traits are required throughout medical school, residency, and the tenure of the career.

I believe it is people who not only have these qualities that make impactful doctors, but also those who pursue medicine ultimately for the service of others. Contributing to this book is important to me because I want to help demystify the process and help students make informed decisions through exploration in the early stages of this career. There is no single, perfect pathway to medicine. People come into the profession with different academic and personal backgrounds, experiences, and skillsets. My hope is this book will help any person, no matter their story, to realize becoming a physician is possible.

Bobbie Ann Adair White

A quick thank you to Rich and Leila for asking me to participate in this advising venture. My career in medical education started in 2004 and continues to this day. Throughout this time, my roles have varied, but the common denominator has always been the students. I have taught, advised, interviewed, and guided students throughout my career. Like Rich and Leila, I have often found that students have not taken the time to self reflect and truly understand what it is that they want from their career.

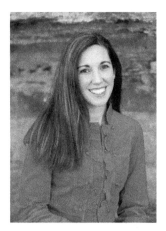

Courtesy Bobbie Ann Adair White

When helping students prepare for their residency application process, I frequently found that they needed to write their statement multiple times and practice their interview questions repetitively to encourage self-reflection, honesty, and vulnerability. Early in my career, I thought it was odd that such multi-talented students were not further along in their self-actualization process, especially because so much of my graduate studies required analytical thinking. However, I have come to the conclusion that the majority of students have not reflected because their grueling educational process does not allow time for self-reflection.

It seems that some students do not start the self-reflection process until they are in their third or fourth year of medical school, which leads to a large amount of anxiety. The third year of medical school is when students are making decisions about residency, and yet some have not narrowed down their interest. This is a more common occurrence than one would think. I have had multiple conversations with students about specialty choice and tried to help them narrow down their options through inquisitive questioning, but nothing is as effective as old-fashioned reflective thinking. It takes time, but it is imperative to helping students make appropriate decisions.

My hope is that this book will help students to critically think about what they want for their future as a whole. What kind of education, practice, lifestyle, and ultimately what kind of professional he or she wants to be. Taking time to review these things will help students persevere and articulate themselves throughout the medical education process.

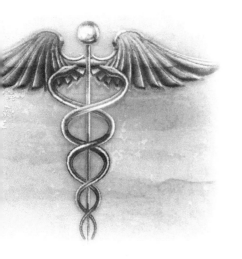

Chapter 1
Guide to Becoming a Physician

It is surprising how few of us understand what a physician specifically does or the education process that is necessary to train a physician in the United States. Yet, thousands of undergraduate students are interested in applying for a chance to join the ranks of health care and to enter medical school.

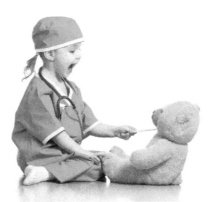

© Oksana Kuzmina, 2014. Used under license from Shutterstock, Inc.

One of the most difficult questions a premedical student will likely be asked is, "Why do you want to become a medical doctor?" Ironically, many premedical students have spent years in their pursuit of a medical career, but struggle to articulate their personal and professional ambitions in both their personal statements and/or professional school interviews. It seems as if they never gave it any significant thought or just took it for granted that they always wanted to be a physician. Some of the most common responses are, "I want to help people." or "I have always loved my science courses." Other students have shared more personal reasons that usually are associated with a tragic or miraculous life event in which the medical professionals deeply affected one of their family members or close friends. Ideally, premedical students will elect to pursue a medical career simply because they appreciate and value the specific responsibilities the physicians will encounter in their everyday practice of medicine.

For many undergraduate students, it is a challenge to discover and to understand the actual responsibilities and expectations of a medical doctor. This could be a result of the many misconceptions about the practice of medicine and the educational training of a physician in the United States. For many years, television and cinema have portrayed medical doctors as extremely intelligent, confident, attractive, and courageous individuals that save the lives of their patients in dramatic and at times, in a heroic fashion. Television always provides wonderful scenes with the doctors demonstrating remarkable skills with fascinating technology at their disposal to restore the life of another individual. Moreover, many of us have some personal memories that focus on the individuals with the white coat and stethoscope who made us feel better or used some interesting technology and gadgets to look into our bodies.

Hospitals seem to be otherworldly and filled with dynamic medical equipment and remarkable individuals in colorful scrubs. It is impossible not to find it fascinating. Unfortunately, this fascination has led to some unrealistic impressions of medicine and the many different professionals involved in treating and caring for the patients. It is easy to get confused and not realize that the medical doctor is but one part of an extensive and complex medical system that we have in the United States.

This text will not attempt to discuss the entire medical profession and its immense corporate and cultural structure. Furthermore, it would be a significant challenge to even explain the multiple dimensions of the roles and responsibilities of the variety of 21st century medical professionals in the United States. Additionally, it will not speculate on the emerging political and economic health care issues that will impact the health professions with the implementation of the Affordable Care Act. Hopefully, your future years of medical training and future undergraduate activities will provide you with the insight to grasp the many political and social aspects of the American health care systems. What this text will discuss is the training process in which a person develops into a capable medical practitioner and some aspects of how research, business, and family will all affect your future ability to serve your patients effectively.

The process to become a licensed medical doctor can be frustratingly mysterious and generally misunderstood. Many people know or have heard about it being a rigorous and grueling ordeal, but few understand how or why. There are many ominous terms that are discussed such as the MCAT, admission statistics, and residency programs, which lead many undergraduates to believe there is some type of "weeding out" process that premedical students must navigate in order to earn a space in a future medical school class. There are courses like Biology, Physics, Organic Chemistry, and Biochemistry that may have some intimidating faculty members that make the premedical curriculum seem overly difficult. In truth, it is challenging to become a medical doctor, but not solely because of the educational process. It may have more to do with the expectations of perfection that we have for physicians and the overall competitiveness of the profession itself. Moreover, the process to become a medical doctor is long, which requires great perseverance and persistence. We all want our medical providers to be capable, competent, compassionate, and intelligent individuals who will make our immediate health concern their top priority through their medical practice.

The medical training process is challenging not only because of the difficult academic material that must be learned, but also because of the many crossroads the future medical provider will face as they advance in their training. There will be many points throughout your education that you will have to make difficult and personal decisions that will certainly affect the rest of your life. In your undergraduate career, as a premedical student, you will have to participate and perform well in select courses and extracurricular activities to be prepared for your future medical training. Then, you will have to complete an extensive application process in which your intellectual skills and personal character will be assessed and measured by medical admission committees. Those fortunate enough to earn a seat in medical school will be again compelled to ingest vast amounts of knowledge through courses and clerkships that will prepare them for their future practice. Along the way, each student will have to choose a medical profession. Each decision takes them on a new and more select pathway in medicine, which will consequently lead to more opportunities for intellectual and personal growth.

Though the text will discuss the many aspects of medicine and the process to become a medical doctor, it would be wise to utilize best sources developed by the Association of American Medical Colleges and the American Association of Colleges of Osteopathic Medicine. Both organizations manage useful and informative websites that allow us to discover the opportunities in medical education and careers in health care. Their websites can be located at www.aamc.org and www.aacom.org. Additionally, students should always engage with their premedical advisors on their college campus as well. They usually have a plethora of resources that can help students discern their professional ambitions.

Student Perspective

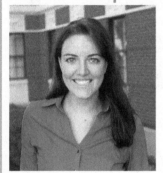

By Jaden Rachel Schupp
Baylor University, 2013; Baylor College of
*   Medicine, 2017*

"Welcome to the profession of medicine." It was the first day of medical school orientation and our Dean of Student Affairs (who is also a remarkable pediatric surgeon and an embryology professor) greeted us with those words. The remaining 40 minutes of her talk focused on and explored the concept of professionalism. Despite the fact that we were only medical students, we were now also medical professionals and we were expected to conduct ourselves as such. In the six months since that time, I have begun to learn what it means to conduct myself as a professional—in social media, in my interactions with my colleagues, and in my interactions with patients. Recently, I was taking the history of a new patient and despite my introduction as a medical student, she continually called me, "Doctor." I'm not ready to bear the full weight and responsibility of that title—but luckily, I have a few more years to prepare before that honorific accurately applies. Many medical schools matriculate their students with some form of a white coat or stethoscope ceremony, formally ushering these new colleagues and physicians in training into the profession, while espousing virtues such as integrity, professionalism, respect, compassion, and self-sacrifice. My question for you is: Are you ready for this? Do you want to enter the profession of medicine?

When I chose to apply for medical school, I didn't have a dramatic story that highlighted my reason to be interested in medicine (I didn't want to be a doctor since I was three, I didn't have a relative who was significantly impacted by a medical professional, I didn't have a single most important shadowing experience that confirmed my interest). But, I knew myself and I knew this was something I wanted to devote myself to pursuing. I would strongly encourage you to spend time reflecting on your interest in medicine as a career (if you "don't have time" to evaluate yourself and your reasons for being pre-med, trust me, your undergraduate years are the most free time you will ever have, if you continue on to medical training—and this is some of the most important thinking you will ever do). Knowing yourself is crucially important to this process. Many times, parents or authority figures put strong pressure on students to pursue medicine, but you must make this choice for yourself. A successful medical

continued

Student Perspective *(continued)*

school application must convince the readers that you know about the life you are signing up for, that you are capable of succeeding, and that you have good reasons for choosing medicine. Time spent now in self-reflection will be invaluable later. And if you decide to no longer be pre-med, that is *okay*—congratulations for knowing yourself and making the right choice for you! If you decide to remain pre-med, write down what you have learned during self-reflection (this will be helpful later when writing application personal statements), and then finish this book. The journey to become a physician is long, arduous, multi-faceted, and rewarding. It is our hope that this book will provide you with the framework and background knowledge necessary for you to be well educated about the medical training process. So keep reading!

Medical school is the hardest thing I have ever done. It is also one of the best. I worked quite tirelessly in my undergraduate years, flourishing in classwork, in extracurricular activities, in leadership positions, in community service activities, and spending numerous hours shadowing (all of these are essential for acceptance into any medical school class). When you enter a medical school class, you will find yourself surrounded by people from all over the country and the world who are as intelligent, accomplished, motivated, and talented as you are, and together you will study and work harder than ever before. But, you will also continue in self-discovery, as you and your classmates discern the field of medicine that you will want to practice. I've had such fun working with physicians in a variety of disciplines, beginning to discover my own medical specialty interests. The time that I get to spend with patients is a wonderful motivator, reminding me of the reasons why I chose to enter the profession of medicine.

Best of luck to you in your own journey towards medicine!

Chapter 1 Worksheet

Why do you want to be a physician?

This is the most important question to ask yourself when you consider becoming a physician. A well-developed response is one that has depth and has been reflected upon for a good time. You should be prepared to answer this question frequently along this pathway.

List below some initial reasons that come to mind for your reason to pursue a career in medicine. Later, you will use these to begin to develop a personal statement for your application to medical school.

1)

2)

3)

4)

5)

6)

7)

List below some reasons or concerns that come to mind that may inhibit your opportunity to become a medical doctor in the future.

1)

2)

3)

4)

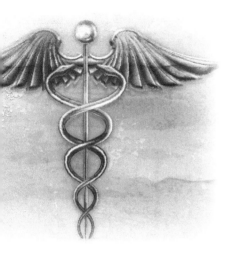

Chapter 2
Undergraduate Premedical Programs

Many students enter college with the intent to one day attend medical school after graduation. To do so, students must undertake series of courses and activities so that they will be eligible to complete an application to any Allopathic or Osteopathic medical school. This chapter will discuss the Medical College Admission Test (MCAT), the curricular

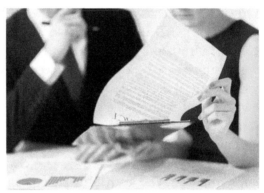

© Syda Productions, 2014. Used under license from Shutterstock, Inc.

requirements, and the extracurricular activities that are necessary to be competitive in the medical school application process.

The Medical College Admission Test (MCAT)

One of the most pertinent criteria utilized by medical colleges' admission committees is the score a student earns on the MCAT. In 2015, the AAMC introduced a new version of the MCAT that was intended to be very different from the previous version. The 2015 MCAT will consequently lead to some modifications in the medical college admission committees' applicant evaluations. Generally, admission committees used the MCAT as a standardized method to compare the intellectual skills of their applicants, which helped them predict which students would be successful in their future medical training. The AAMC intends to have the 2015 version of the MCAT provide more substantial information about the applicant's ability to manage the complex medical and physiological issues they will encounter in a medical career. Students can visit the website https://www.aamc.org/students/applying/mcat to learn more about the 2015 MCAT.

The MCAT has four distinct sections: Biological and Biochemical Foundations of Living Systems, Chemical and Physical Foundations of Biological Systems, Psychological, Social and Biological Foundations of Behavior, and

Critical Analysis and Reasoning Skills. Consequently, the academic content of the MCAT will include material from Biology, Inorganic (General) Chemistry, Organic Chemistry, Biochemistry, Physics, Psychology, and Sociology. Though there are not specific mathematical topics on the MCAT, it will be helpful to have a background in calculus and statistics. It is not necessary or required to participate in formal coursework in these academic areas to take the MCAT, but a student will certainly be at a disadvantage without the appropriate academic preparation.

Naturally, the MCAT and its value in the medical school admission process will lead to some anxiety for premedical students, but there are many opportunities and methods to prepare for it. Several commercial programs offer formal test preparation for the MCAT and these can be a good option for some students. Other students choose to study for the MCAT on their own, using a variety of published MCAT preparation books, in lieu of paying for and attending a formal course. In truth, the best method to prepare for the MCAT is to take full advantage of the coursework in your undergraduate career. The MCAT will measure your working knowledge of the sciences and social sciences, and the more knowledgeable and comfortable you are with these subjects, the greater success you should have. The MCAT is remarkably challenging and you will need to develop a strategy to best prepare for it. To do so, a student should diligently and intentionally take time to visit the MCAT website **https://www.aamc.org/students/applying/mcat/** and learn as much as possible about the exam. AAMC provides an opportunity for students to take a free practice MCAT, in addition to providing some great advice to be better prepared for the test. Additional practice examinations are offered by the AAMC, but are not free. These practice tests are an excellent means to assess your preparation and readiness for the exam.

Getting accustomed to a standardized test like the MCAT is a challenge for nearly every premedical student. The 2015 MCAT will attempt to measure your critical reasoning skills as well as your knowledge of the basic sciences and social sciences. It stands to reason that all students should take efforts throughout their undergraduate career to improve their abilities in the particular MCAT subject areas. Being diligent and working hard in your undergraduate coursework will certainly improve your readiness for the MCAT. Many premedical students elect to take additional biological coursework in order to better prepare for the subject material for the MCAT. But, since only a quarter of the subject matter of the MCAT focuses on biological material, this approach may not necessarily provide the advantages the premedical student is seeking. Pursuing a balanced curriculum, while taking the suggested courses for the MCAT, will certainly prepare all students for the content to be tested on the MCAT.

Many students overlook the value of developing their critical reasoning and reading skills for the MCAT and spend too much effort focusing on the sciences. The Critical Reasoning and the Social Behavior sections comprise one-half of the total MCAT score. Consequently, pursuing a well-rounded curriculum with the intent to development critical reasoning skills is encouraged. Moreover, students should make an effort to exercise their reading skills and develop their ability to comprehend a variety of material. Taking time to read outside of the classroom (but not at the expense of success in classwork) will certainly be helpful in preparing.

Table 2-1: MCAT Scores and GPAs for Applicants and Matriculants to U.S. Medical Schools, 2002–2013

Average MCAT scores and GPAs for applicants and matriculants are displayed below. Please e-mail us at datarequest@aamc.org if you need further assistance or have additional inquiries.

Applicants		2002	2003	2004	2005	2006	2007	2008	2009	2010	2011	2012	2013
MCAT VR	Mean	8.7	8.6	8.9	8.9	8.9	9.0	9.0	9.0	9.1	9.0	9.0	9.1
	SD*	2.2	2.2	2.2	2.2	2.2	2.3	2.2	2.2	2.1	2.1	2.1	2.2
MCAT PS	Mean	9.0	8.9	8.9	9.0	9.0	9.2	9.3	9.2	9.4	9.4	9.5	9.5
	SD	2.2	2.2	2.2	2.2	2.3	2.3	2.3	2.3	2.3	2.3	2.3	2.3
MCAT BS	Mean	9.3	9.2	9.3	9.4	9.5	9.6	9.8	9.8	9.8	9.9	9.9	9.8
	SD	2.1	2.1	2.1	2.1	2.1	2.2	2.1	2.2	2.1	2.1	2.1	2.1
Total MCAT	Mean	27.0	26.8	27.1	27.3	27.4	27.7	28.1	27.9	28.3	28.2	28.3	28.4
	SD	5.6	5.6	5.5	5.6	5.6	5.8	5.6	5.6	5.5	5.5	5.5	5.5
MCAT WS	Median	O	P	O	O	O	O	P	O	P	P	P	P
GPA Science	Mean	3.36	3.36	3.36	3.37	3.38	3.39	3.40	3.41	3.43	3.43	3.44	3.44
	SD	0.46	0.46	0.46	0.45	0.45	0.45	0.44	0.44	0.43	0.43	0.43	0.43
GPA Non-Science	Mean	3.59	3.60	3.60	3.60	3.61	3.62	3.63	3.64	3.65	3.65	3.66	3.66
	SD	0.34	0.33	0.33	0.32	0.32	0.32	0.31	0.31	0.30	0.30	0.31	0.30
GPA Total	Mean	3.46	3.47	3.47	3.48	3.48	3.49	3.50	3.51	3.53	3.53	3.54	3.54
	SD	0.37	0.37	0.37	0.36	0.37	0.36	0.36	0.35	0.35	0.34	0.34	0.34
Total Applicants		*33,624*	*34,791*	*35,735*	*37,372*	*39,108*	*42,315*	*42,231*	*42,268*	*42,741*	*43,919*	*45,266*	*48,014*

Matriculants		2002	2003	2004	2005	2006	2007	2008	2009	2010	2011	2012	2013
MCAT VR	Mean	9.5	9.5	9.7	9.7	9.8	9.9	9.9	9.8	9.9	9.8	9.8	10.0
	SD	1.8	1.7	1.7	1.8	1.7	1.8	1.8	1.7	1.7	1.7	1.7	1.7
MCAT PS	Mean	10.0	9.9	9.9	10.0	10.1	10.3	10.3	10.3	10.4	10.4	10.5	10.6
	SD	1.9	1.9	1.9	1.9	1.9	1.9	2.0	2.0	1.9	1.9	1.9	1.9
MCAT BS	Mean	10.2	10.2	10.3	10.4	10.5	10.6	10.7	10.8	10.8	10.8	10.9	10.8
	SD	1.6	1.6	1.6	1.6	1.6	1.7	1.7	1.7	1.7	1.6	1.6	1.6
Total MCAT	Mean	29.6	29.6	29.9	30.2	30.3	30.8	30.9	30.8	31.1	31.1	31.2	31.3
	SD	4.3	4.2	4.1	4.3	4.2	4.2	4.2	4.1	4.1	4.1	4.0	4.0
MCAT WS	Median	P	P	P	P	P	P	P	P	Q	Q	Q	Q
GPA Science	Mean	3.54	3.55	3.56	3.56	3.57	3.59	3.60	3.60	3.61	3.61	3.63	3.63
	SD	0.36	0.35	0.35	0.35	0.34	0.33	0.33	0.32	0.32	0.32	0.31	0.31
GPA Non-Science	Mean	3.69	3.70	3.70	3.70	3.71	3.73	3.73	3.74	3.75	3.74	3.75	3.76
	SD	0.27	0.26	0.26	0.27	0.26	0.25	0.25	0.25	0.24	0.25	0.24	0.23
GPA Total	Mean	3.61	3.62	3.62	3.63	3.64	3.65	3.66	3.66	3.67	3.67	3.68	3.69
	SD	0.29	0.28	0.28	0.28	0.27	0.27	0.26	0.26	0.26	0.26	0.25	0.25
Total Matriculants		*16,488*	*16,541*	*16,648*	*17,003*	*17,361*	*17,759*	*18,036*	*18,390*	*18,665*	*19,230*	*19,517*	*20,055*

* SD = Standard Deviation

Source: AAMC 12/5/2013

As mentioned previously, the 2015 will have four distinct sections that will each be individually scored. The scores for each section can range from 118 to 132 with the score of 125 being the median or midpoint. The examinees will also be given a percentile rank for each section as well, which will likely be used as a measurement by the medical school admission committees as well. The sections scores will then be tallied for a combined score, which will range from 472 to 528 with 500 being the median or midpoint. In addition to the composite score, the MCAT will also provide an overall percentile rank that will tell you how you compared to all the other MCAT examinees.

To be competitive in the medical school application cycle, students will want to earn the highest possible scores within each MCAT subsection. It will likely be detrimental to your medical school application if one or more of the subsection scores are below the median score of 125. Moreover, students will want to achieve a composite score of 500 or greater to be competitive in the medical school admission cycle. In Table 2-1 the previous MCAT scores and ranks have been provided to give some indication on the competitiveness of the medical school admission process and the general scores needed by students in the past to successfully matriculate into medical school. The percentile rank that will now be provided with the overall composite score has not been a factor for medical school admission committees in the past, but it will likely be used in the future. Consequently, medical school applicants will need to be aware of their percentile scores as well as their composite scores. It is important to note that the MCAT composite score and percentile rank will not be the only variables considered by the medical school admission committee, but they certainly will effect your overall competitiveness in the application process.

The MCAT is a computerized test and is offered from the months of January through September. Technically, students can take the test as often as they would like, but it is generally recommended that they should not take the MCAT more than three times. Typically, students will take their first MCAT in the spring semester of their 3rd (Junior) year; however, the date on which a student selects to take the MCAT will vary depending on the student's academic program. It is important that MCAT studying/preparing is given sufficient time, but it must also be balanced with the courses in which a student is enrolled. Poor classroom performance, and a subsequent decrease in GPA, is not excused by MCAT preparation. Conversely, inadequate MCAT preparation due to a demanding course load and other commitments is also something to avoid. Students should not take their first MCAT until they feel ready—luck will never be a factor when taking the MCAT. Readiness is easily gauged by taking some of the many practice MCAT tests that exist online and consistently earning the desired score range.

The Premedical Course Curriculum

Application to a US Medical School/College requires completion of a specific curriculum. Much of the premedical curriculum is established as a consequence of MCAT material; however, there are several additional courses that most medical schools require to complete an application.

Some colleges/universities may have a premedical major that will incorporate all the courses necessary for medical school, but most academic institutions will simply blend the coursework into traditional academic programs such as Biology or Chemistry. When considering the coursework in a premedical program, students must take care in selecting their undergraduate major/academic program. There always seems to be discussion as to what is the best major to be competitive for medical school. The truth is, no specific academic major/program is better than any other in helping a student become a successful medical doctor. Students should consider how to incorporate necessary premedical coursework into the required coursework of their chosen academic program. Often, students will major in Biology, Biochemistry, Chemistry, or another science because the premedical requirements are already satisfied by the requirements of their major. However, it is not rare to find students in a medical school class who majored in the social sciences, business or the arts, but they took efforts to ensure that they could also include the required premedical courses via electives or summer school. If this is not feasible, you may want to discuss with your academic advisor about other options.

At this time, many medical schools require a variety of courses, but there has been some review and consideration as to which courses best prepare a student for a career as a medical doctor. The recent trend for medical education is to focus on competency in specific areas. You can refer to the following website about the list of competencies many medical schools will be seeking in the future: **https://www.aamc.org/initiatives/admissionsinitiative/competencies /#.UrjZMZUWGkg**. Competency is much more challenging for medical school admission boards to measure, but students will need to begin demonstrating an ability to *use* the knowledge they attain in their coursework.

Students should thoroughly investigate every medical school to which they plan to apply. Many medical schools may require additional coursework in the sciences, humanities, or social sciences, including some of the recommended courses listed in the table. Many of the courses listed in the table may also be knowledge tested on the MCAT examination, so they are *strongly* recommended so that premedical students are better prepared for this examination.

Many premedical students are likely to have earned credit for some of the courses listed in the table while attending high school via AP/IB credit or dual credit. It is debatable whether or not students need to repeat these courses for medical school. There are a significant number of medical schools that prefer all of these courses be taken during the student's traditional undergraduate career, but very few if any have made it a requirement. Consequently, it is up to each individual to determine the best course of action for his or her undergraduate career. Introductory courses in Biology and Chemistry are generally the foundation of advanced coursework like Genetics and Biochemistry. If the coursework undertaken in high school is subpar, students may struggle in their advanced science coursework as a result. Therefore, many premedical advisors encourage students to evaluate their high school work and repeat the coursework during their undergraduate career if necessary.

Course	Credit Hours	Required/ Recommended
Intro Biology	8 Hours (2 Hours of Lab)	Required
Chemistry	8 Hours (2 Hours of Lab)	Required
Physics	8 Hours (2 Hours of Lab)	Required
Organic Chemistry	8 Hours (2 Hours of Lab)	Required
Biochemistry	3–4 Hours (Lab Optional)	Required
Genetics	3–4 Hours (Lab Optional)	Recommended
English Composition	6 Hours	Required
Psychology	3 Hours	Recommended (MCAT)
Sociology	3 Hours	Recommended (MCAT)
Calculus	3–4 Hours	Required
Statistics	3–4 Hours	Highly Recommended

It is generally recommended that students complete all these courses before they take the MCAT examination and apply to medical school, but there are exceptions to this advice. Technically, students can take the MCAT at any time and are not required to have the coursework completed beforehand. Moreover, students can apply to medical school without the coursework completed as well. Most medical schools will still consider the application, but will require that the coursework be completed before they will officially admit the applicant.

In the following chapters, we will discuss the application process and how medical schools will evaluate your readiness for medical training. It will not be enough to simply take the required coursework.

Extracurricular Activities and Medical Exploration

Shadowing

It has become a basic expectation that students attain some professional shadowing experience during their undergraduate career. The medical application process only allows activities from the undergraduate career to be recognized, so any shadowing completed during high school will not be considered. Unfortunately, shadowing can be very difficult to attain. A federal law known as HIPAA (http://www.hhs.gov/ocr/privacy/) protects the privacy of patients, and consequently makes your participation in shadowing a liability for many medical doctors and their practice. If a shadowing student ever revealed confidential and protected patient information, the physician/medical center would be held responsible. Therefore, many hospitals and medical doctors do not facilitate the opportunity for undergraduates to shadow. It requires a great deal of trust in the student for a physician to allow their presence in the room with a patient.

To attain the opportunity to shadow, it is ideal to develop a relationship with a physician that you already know. If possible, begin with a family member or close family friend who works the health care industry. If there are no relatives, the next option would be the your own family physician or health care provider. If neither of these are viable options, students can always solicit physicians in the local area of their school or near their home. Remember, trust will have to be established between you and the physician. To establish this trust, a student must present himself or herself as a conscientious and responsible adult. It would be wise to create a résumé of your education and experiences that you can send to physicians for potential shadowing. The résumé should be accompanied with a cover letter explaining your intention to acquire shadowing experience in their practice. If you have previous shadowing experience from high school and/or HIPAA training, include this in the résumé. If you pursue this route, it is unlikely that the first physician you approach will accept you as a shadowing student. It is challenging to find a willing physician, so it is recommended that you begin the search early. Be aware of area saturation—successfully approaching a physician is difficult given the high number of premedical students in college looking for the same opportunity. It is not impossible, but you will have to make a strong case for yourself. Instead, approaching physicians in your hometown for summer shadowing can often be more successful. In order to set up a summer shadowing opportunity, it is encouraged to begin your ef-

forts over Christmas break and during the spring semester—it can take a few months to put everything in place, and starting in April or May will often result in an unsuccessful search. Despite the difficulty of orchestrating shadowing, the opportunity will be well worth it—direct experience with actual medicine and patients is invaluable.

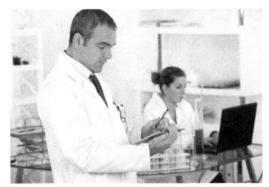

© auremar, 2014. Used under license from Shutterstock, Inc.

Many osteopathic medical schools will require shadowing experience with an osteopathic physician before they will consider your application for admission. More often than not, the osteopathic medical schools will also seek a letter of support from these physicians as well. Therefore, you need to ensure that the experience demonstrates your diligence and interest in the osteopathic profession.

Regardless if you are shadowing an osteopathic or allopathic physician, you want to be prepared for and to make the most of the experience. There is little that you will be able to do to help or assist the physician during the day, so do not worry about having any specific skills or abilities. The best way to prepare for the shadowing experience is to learn as much as possible about the physician that will be followed. If you can discover information about their medical practice and their medical training, you will know what you will likely encounter during the day. Asking good questions and demonstrating your interest in medicine is easily the best way to impress the physician. Show them that you are serious about learning and demonstrate a genuine respect for the medical profession. However, if the physician or surgeon is in the middle of a procedure or examination, it is best to keep quiet unless you are invited to ask questions. A good shadow is a *shadow* that knows how to ask good questions at appropriate times.

There is no specific time requirement for shadowing. The general expectation is about 50 hours, but each student should determine the amount of time that they need to understand the medical profession. It is good to have a variety of experiences if possible, and the more a student shadows the more they will generally know about medicine. Therefore, students are encouraged to shadow as much as they are able.

Student Organizations/Extracurricular Activities

Medical school admission boards will always seek extracurricular experiences in the applications of the students. How a student spends his or her time outside of the classroom conveys a great deal about the student's values and interests. Therefore, premedical students need to be considerate and intentional of the activities they elect to pursue during their undergraduate career.

All student organizations and extracurricular activities certainly have their benefits and can develop many wonderful attributes that will help students become better medical doctors. When selecting activities, premedical students need to consider several factors. What is the time commitment? What are the requirements for participation? What skills will be gained by participation in this activity? If the activity or organization impedes on your academic progress and success, then you have to determine if the skills and attributes gained from the experiences are worth the additional stress in your undergraduate career. At no point should grades be sacrificed to participate in extracurricular activities.

Medical schools value many different attributes besides the traditional academic abilities demonstrated in the classroom (medical schools' admission processes will be discussed in the next chapter). Students can use extracurricular activities to demonstrate skills in leadership and research. Student organizations allow students to demonstrate social skills like compassion and empathy. A successful physician or surgeon has to be able to interact with a variety of personalities and be aware of the many cultural concerns that their patients will bring into the examination room. Student organizations are a great means to interact with others and develop the extraverted abilities for a medical career.

If the university/college offers them, student organizations that focus on the health profession are great options for premedical students. They can provide opportunities for students to interact with a variety of medical professionals and other premedical undergraduates. Many of these organizations provide opportunities for shadowing experiences and other medically related activities. Moreover, it is always beneficial to interact with upperclassmen that are further along in their premedical preparation and gain insight from their experiences. Most importantly, participating in pre-health-related student organizations will demonstrate your interest in the medical professions. Medical schools appreciate any demonstrated interest in medicine and there is no easier method to accomplish this.

Ultimately, when selecting an activity or student organization, you should select those opportunities that you most enjoy and fit your specific interests. You will always be most successful in activities that you genuinely enjoy.

Community Service

As mentioned earlier, medical school admission boards greatly appreciate when applicants demonstrate compassion and empathy in their undergraduate activities. Participation in community service activities is advantageous. There are actually multiple forms of community service, and students need to be thoughtful in considering which community service activities would be most beneficial.

There are three general types of health-related community service in which undergraduates can participate: medical mission trips, continuous service activities, and one-time service events. These community service experiences all have their benefits and drawbacks.

Medical mission trips generally require the participation of certified medical professionals. There are some organizations such as International Service Learning (http://www.islonline.org) or Unite for Sight (http://www.unitefor sight.org) that coordinate individual medical mission trips for undergraduate students. Some student organizations on your campus may be able to provide these international experiences as well. Medical mission trips are expensive and can be dangerous, depending on the location. Nevertheless, students can have terrific experiences and learn a great deal about medicine by working in these settings.

Continuous service experiences are generally the best community service experiences that students can have. It is an excellent method to demonstrate your commitment to a specific cause or interest. A student can cultivate particular skills and abilities through a continuous service program as well. For medical school admission, it would be ideal if these service projects were at health-related sites like clinics, nursing facilities, hospitals, or health-related organizations. Tutoring programs at local schools are also great opportunities to demonstrate academic skills and a value for education. These types of services programs require an extensive commitment from the students and could be difficult to maintain with a rigorous academic curriculum. Short-term summer volunteer programs are an alternative to manage this concern.

One-time service events are great opportunities to participate in meaningful activities and demonstrate compassion and civic-mindedness. Many college campuses and student organizations sponsor these events throughout the academic year. Relay-For-Life is a great example of a one-time service event that can have a great benefit for the medical community. These activities are easy to manage with a challenging semester of coursework. Unfortunately, the events do not allow for any development of skills or significant personal attributes. Nevertheless, these one-time service events are certainly better than not participating in service at all.

Undergraduate Research

Research is the cornerstone of science and of medicine. It does not mean that every physician or surgeon should be capable of conducting research, but an excellent health care provider should be able to read and understand the emerging literature. Consequently, medical school admission committees have begun to seek this ability in their applicants.

We will discuss medical research in greater detail in Chapter 12. While a crucial aspect of the premedical undergraduate career, it seems to be misunderstood. Undergraduates do not need to participate in an undergraduate research experience to be competitive for medical school admission, but the experience is advantageous for their future application.

The AAMC has a useful link for students seeking undergraduate research opportunities during the summer: **https://www.aamc.org/members/great/ 61052/great_summerlinks.html**. The list of medical schools providing undergraduate research programs is very extensive and many of these programs have the funding to pay the students over the summer for their efforts. These programs are competitive, so students should plan on applying to multiple programs. It is important that students begin their investigation of potential programs in the fall semester—many applications are due in early January or February and compiling a competitive application and obtaining letters of recommendation take time.

Attaining opportunities to participate in undergraduate research at one's home university can be challenging. Students need to be persistent and diligent in investigating their college's resources about professors who need support for their research projects and laboratories. Investigating the research in a laboratory is important before approaching a professor about working with them. Faculty members recognize achievement in the classroom as well as in the laboratories that coincide with their courses. Therefore, students need to focus on their performance in the classroom so they can be competitive for research opportunities.

Attaining Letters of Recommendation from the Faculty

One of the most challenging and often overlooked aspects of a successful undergraduate career is the attainment of letters of recommendation from the faculty. Any undergraduate planning on applying to medical school will need letters from multiple faculty members, particularly professors from the sciences. This can be even more challenging at large universities and colleges that host heavily populated courses. Even if a student does well in the class, there is a good possibility that they may have rarely spoken to the professor.

Premedical students have to make a conscientious effort to engage with their professors. This can be easily achieved by effectively utilizing office hours. Asking thoughtful and insightful questions during office hours is a great way to demonstrate interest in learning the subject material. There may be other activities in which you can interact with your professors, such as honor societies, undergraduate research, and other departmental events. It is wise to invest some time and effort to participate in your major so that professors can witness your maturity and abilities outside of the classroom. It is crucial to remember that every interaction you have with a professor is a time that they may be evaluating you. Dressing well, behaving maturely, paying attention during class (rather than being distracted by your phone or computer), doing well on exams, and talking to the professor before or after class can be good ways to make a good impression on a professor. A good letter of recommendation doesn't come from someone who remembers you as the sloppy jerk who was repeatedly tardy and failed a test. Additionally, when talking to professors, remember that they are extremely busy, and it is important to be respectful of their time. Students should make an effort in each of their classes to make sure that the professor knows him or her, and these efforts should begin in the first year. Don't wait until you start applying to make contacts with your professors. The more the faculty who are able to share in a letter of support, the more effective one's letters will be in the medical school application process.

Final Thoughts

Navigating the premedical requirements as an undergraduate is certainly challenging and will require diligence and great effort. Hopefully, you will enjoy many of the classes and extracurricular activities. As you will learn in the next chapter, premedical students do not have to be perfect to successfully enter medical school, but it is a competitive process. Spend your time wisely and invest your efforts into activities and studies that will cultivate the abilities and background you may need to be successful in your future medical career. Give your decision about becoming a medical doctor some serious thought and take the time to explore your professional aspirations through shadowing and extracurricular activities.

Student Perspective

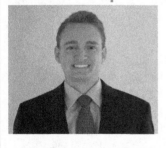

By Dustin Luse
Baylor University, 2014

If you had asked me why I wanted to be a doctor during each year of undergrad, you would have gotten at least four different answers. I was sure I wanted to be a surgeon freshman year, because the thrill of being in the operating room and working with my hands was very appealing, so I pursued no fewer than ten surgical shadowing opportunities during college. As I observed the patient-physician relationship among most surgeons, I sensed their interactions were often cold and mechanical, devoid of the pleasant and seemingly friendly communication of primary care doctors, who develop closer relationships with their patients because of regular visits.

These experiences led me to question my ambition to become a surgeon and I explored other areas of medicine through shadowing and service because of my desire to build lasting relationships with patients. I joined the Multicultural Association of Prehealth Students and attended medical mission trips to Panama and the Dominican Republic in an effort to gain a better understanding of other cultures and how their values, beliefs, and perceptions influence communication and relationships with health

continued

Student Perspective *(continued)*

care providers. I began to apply what I was learning by practicing my communication skills and bedside manner with terminally ill patients at a local hospice service. Through these encounters, I became passionate about optimizing the patient experience and working to eliminate many of the inequalities in the US health care system. I chose to major in Economics instead of Biology or Chemistry because I wanted to understand the mechanisms behind the delivery of health care services and acquire the skills and knowledge to make a difference on a larger scale.

A medical school interviewer once told me it is important to keep an open mind during undergraduate and medical education and not to be disappointed in yourself if your career aspirations change because that is the essence of learning. He compared college to Earth and medical school to Mars, and said you can't really know what it is like or what you want to do until you are actually there, experiencing things first-hand.

Undergrad education serves as a launching point where you have the opportunity to learn about why you want to go on this journey but you don't know quite where it will take you. A good medical school applicant is someone who explores different areas of interest, meets new people, takes risks, and makes mistakes; all while reflecting continuously on why they are pursuing medicine and how their experiences are shaping them into the kind of doctor patients want to see. So why not consider a new major or minor; go abroad to study or serve; join a unique organization or club; make friends who are different from you; and serve in as many ways as you can. You never know what you might learn about yourself and how it will help you tell your story to your future medical school.

Gerardo Martinez

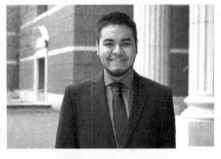

University of Texas Southwestern Medical Student Class of 2019

I didn't always know I wanted to go into medicine. I didn't know I wanted to be a doctor since I was three, I didn't have a calling, I didn't have a eureka moment from which my passion arose, nor did I know what actual medicine entailed. As I stood there on my first day of freshman year, I had a desire to learn, a backpack filled with hopes, and a nervous feeling in my stomach.

The first year of undergrad I spent trying to figure out exactly what I wanted to pursue. I loaded my courses with the basics and tried to ask as many questions as possible. I joined a variety of organizations ranging from medical oriented groups like AMSA all the way to cultural groups like HSA to try to learn more about what I enjoyed.

After acclimating to the college environment during my second year I took a decisive step in my future and decided to apply to Alpha Epsilon Delta. It was through this organization that I had the opportunity to grow beyond the confines of what could be learned through studying. It was the opportunity to learn by doing and I took a hold of everything I could get my hands on. This included serving as a volunteer at the Family Health Center on South 18 where I was given the chance to learn about what goes on to provide effective care to the Waco residents behind the front desk, behind the nurses' station, and in a physician's shadow. I was able to form what I believed it meant to truly serve another human being by shadowing the doctors who demonstrated selfless devotion to those who entrusted them with their care.

My passion for service was given a chance to develop, but my academic drive was also allowed to go beyond the books. After serving as a lab assistant for human physiology for a year, I was able to develop a relationship with the lab coordinator. From this relationship, I was given the chance to demonstrate my drive for science and my desire to learn more than what was taught. Our conversations about the lab coordinators research on zebrafish soon turned into discussions about what they were currently working on and finally a chance to work on a project under them. Research is difficult, it is time consuming, repetitive, frustrating, but it is also fulfilling.

The same person that stood nervously on the first day of college was also the same person that worked to learn more, grow as a person, and serve others. Undergrad is a time to search for what makes people wake up for every morning. Whether that be waking up with the goal to serve as many people as possible, waking up to do more than what was done yesterday, or simply waking up to learn more about everything. This is the time to make mistakes, take chances, and go with what you feel is right. Don't be afraid to fail or be afraid of uncertainty, instead embrace them as who you are and grow from them. If you are unsure about what motivates you, take every chance you can get to explore every aspect of what drew you to medicine. Was it the service, the intellectual stimulation, or the chance to make a difference? The most important thing to remember, don't be afraid to be yourself after all you're the one who wants to someday be a physician.

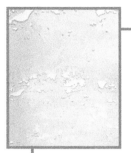

Chapter 2 Worksheet

Goals

Create a list of goals to achieve during undergraduate school that will prepare you to become a competitive applicant for medical school. Indicate when you realistically plan to achieve each one by.

1)

2)

3)

4)

5)

6)

7)

Which of these goals will be the most challenging and what is your plan to ensure its success?

What are the specific premedical extracurricular activities that best suit your personal interests?

What are the specific premedical courses that you consider to be most difficult? What is your plan to ensure your success in these specific courses?

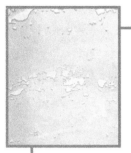

Pick two medical schools that would be at the top of your list to attend. Review their websites and answer the following:

What basis did you use to select these two?

What are their goals (review their mission/vision statements)?

    1)

    2)

What makes them stand out?

After reviewing their websites, would they still be in your top two (why/why not)?

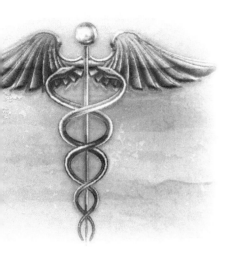

Chapter 3
Medical School Application Process

The decision to apply to medical school comes about for many different reasons. Some say they have wanted to be a doctor since childhood, while others say they decided when they took science courses and became intrigued with all the body entails. Regardless of how or why the decision was made to pursue a career as a physician, there are many actions to be taken to demonstrate one's

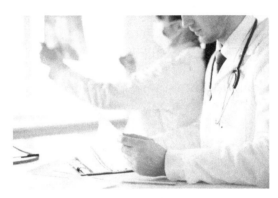

© Syda Productions, 2014. Used under license from Shutterstock, Inc.

passion for medicine. One of first gateways to fulfilling this dream will be to apply to medical school. The application process is very detailed and lengthy and requires planning to submit the best application.

Research Schools to see best for you

Just before applying to medical school, it is a good idea for applicants to research the medical schools they think they are interested in and those not previously considered. If the opportunity presents itself, a visit to the school for a tour or presentation to learn more about the program will help the applicant get a feel for the environment and enhance the knowledge of whether the program would be a fit.

The mission and vision statements of the medical schools should be reviewed as they provide an overview of what is important to that institution. This helps determine if the school matches an applicant's interests, philosophy toward education, and priorities.

If an applicant has a specific interest in primary care, rural medicine, or other areas, he/she will find a better fit with schools that serve those interests. Some medical schools will provide tracks or programs of interest in specific areas.

Schools will often publish data on their matriculated classes on their websites. This will give applicants an indication of how they might fit in or if they will be considered competitive. Broader data on matriculants can be found through the Association of American Medical Colleges' (AAMC) website at www.aamc.org/facts or the Texas Medical and Dental Schools Application Service (TMDSAS) at www.tmdsas.com/medical/application-statistics.html.

Application Services

*3 application services

When applicants are considering which medical schools they intend on applying to, they need to be aware that there are three application services in the nation. The Texas Medical and Dental Schools Application Service (TMDSAS) handles the applications for 10 out of 11 Texas medical schools, the American Medical College Application Service (AMCAS) handles the remaining MD programs in the nation, and the American Association of Colleges of Osteopathic Medicine Application Service (AACOMAS) handles the majority of the DO applications. TMDSAS, AMCAS, and AACOMAS all open for applications in early May, but have differing deadline dates, sometimes down to each school, especially if applicants are applying to special programs.

Each of the application services requires payment to apply. It is important to read each website to understand how cost is determined, how payment is made, and when it is due. In most cases, not submitting payment results in an incomplete application or an application not being processed.

TMDSAS

The Texas Medical and Dental Schools Application Service is the application service for the public medical schools in Texas. As of 2014, there are 11 medical schools in Texas, 10 of which are public schools. The public schools include:

- Texas A&M Health Science Center College of Medicine
- Texas Tech Health Sciences Center School of Medicine
- Texas Tech Health Sciences Center Paul L. Foster School of Medicine
- University of North Texas Health Science Center, Texas College of Osteopathic Medicine
- University of Texas Dell Medical School
- University of Texas Rio Grande Valley School of Medicine
- University of Texas Health Science Center at Houston Medical School
- University of Texas Medical Branch at Galveston
- University of Texas School of Medicine at San Antonio
- University of Texas Southwestern Medical Center

TMDSAS has its own application timeline and process. Applicants should review the entire website to ensure they are following the correct process when applying to these Texas schools. The TMDSAS website is: http://www.tmdsas.com/medical/homepage.html. The application opens May 1st with an October 1st deadline.

There is one private medical school in Texas that does not use TMDSAS —Baylor College of Medicine (BCM). Applicants who wish to apply to BCM as well as to other non-Texas MD schools, must submit an AMCAS application or AACOMAS application for DO schools.

AMCAS

The American Medical College Application Service is the national application service for all MD programs outside of the Texas schools that use TMDSAS. AMCAS falls under the AAMC umbrella. The AMCAS website is: https://www.aamc.org/students/applying/amcas/. AMCAS schools have different deadlines, some into the spring.

AACOMAS

Applicants wishing to apply to DO programs (osteopathic medical schools) can do so through the American Association of Colleges of Osteopathic Medicine Application Service. The AACOMAS website is: http://www.aacom.org/become-a-doctor/applying. The only DO school that does not utilize AACOMAS is the University of North Texas Health Science Center Texas College of Osteopathic Medicine, which uses TMDSAS. Similar to AMCAS schools, AACOMAS schools have different deadlines. Osteopathic medicine is described further in *Chapter 5: Osteopathic Medicine and Allopathic Medicine.*

Secondary (Supplemental) Applications

Several medical schools also have a required or optional secondary or supplemental application. These applications also have deadline dates. Schools that require a secondary application may not review a primary application if the secondary application has not been submitted. Other schools provide it as an optional component.

These applications are typically shorter and are used to gather additional information about the applicant that is specific to the school's mission/vision and their programs. They may also be used to gather additional demographic information (e.g., if the applicant grew up in a medically underserved area), inquire about any specific interests in medicine, or allow the applicant to indicate if he/she is interested in the offered dual degrees at that school.

There may be different processes for how to complete a secondary application. Visit each school's website to determine that process. In most cases, applicants will complete the applications via the school's website. Additionally, some schools may "invite" or ask applicants to complete a secondary application after an initial screening of the primary application and as a continuation in the process. Other schools provide it as an open application for all to complete. In that case, it can be freely accessed on the school's website. These can be completed and submitted independent of the primary application.

Some schools charge a fee for submitting a secondary application. Often, if this payment is not received, the application is not considered complete.

The TMDSAS schools that require secondary applications and their deadlines can be found at the following website: http://www.tmdsas.com/medical/application-instructions.html#sec_application.

The AACOMAS supplemental deadline dates for each DO medical school can be found at the following website: www.aacom.org/news-and-events/publications/cib

Each of the AMCAS schools' websites should be visited to determine if there is a secondary application and the deadline dates.

International Applicants

Aspiring physicians who are not US citizens or US Permanent Residents should contact the schools they are interested in about whether they accept international students. Most medical schools will publish this information on their websites. Some schools will accept Deferred Action for Childhood Arrivals (DACA) applicants, while others do not.

Letters of Recommendation/Evaluation

Letters provide an important perspective on the applicant. They give insight from various experiences. They can also serve to provide insight into potential weaknesses or concerns. Ultimately, they provide an assessment and level of support (usually on a scale) regarding the applicant's suitability to succeed in medical school and beyond.

Recommendation vs. Evaluation Letters

There is a difference between letters of recommendation and letters of evaluation. Letters of recommendation are typically favorable and supportive of the applicant and highlight the activities in which the applicant has been involved, provide examples of observations and interactions with the applicant, and end with a statement about the level of support of the applicant. In essence, they accomplish just as they describe: "recommending" the applicant to medical school.

A letter of evaluation may be more involved and in addition to strengths may also provide insight about weaknesses. Rather than recounting the activities already found in the application, an evaluation letter may provide assessments of the applicant's work in the classroom, lab, work setting, etc. They may provide details of observed difficulties the applicant has had in these settings, accounts of professionalism issues, and/or how prepared the applicant may be to move on to the next stage—medical school. At the end of the letter, applicants are often ranked as compared to their peers (i.e., upper 15%).

Health Professions Packet

Some application processes may allow for more letters to be submitted if a health professions packet is used. Some colleges/universities have an involved health professions office that may provide these packets while others may not. There are different ways packets are submitted so it will be important to check with the health professions office/advisor on the policies and procedures.

A packet may contain several letters from various people including professors, employment supervisors, people with whom the applicant has volunteered, or research mentors, just to name a few. The packet may simply include all of the letters with a cover letter from the health professions office acknowledging the letters as a packet.

If an institution has a dedicated health professions office/advisor and staffing to handle the number of yearly medical applicants, they may be able to provide more involved services. If this is the case, the health professions advisor may write a summary letter based on interaction or an interview with the applicant and attach it along with the other letters. In contrast, other advisors may use information from the submitted letters and quote or summarize them in an overview letter, submitting this alone rather than attaching the original letters.

Applicants should explore early whether their college/university has a health professions office that offers a health professions packet, and follow the procedures outlined by the office to obtain one.

Individual Letters

If the college/university does not have a health professions office/advisor that collects and submits packets on the applicant's behalf or the applicant chooses not to use this resource, individual letters of recommendation should be submitted. Applicants should be careful to review the application instructions to verify how many letters should be submitted.

Some medical schools may require letters from people in certain roles, so instructions should be read carefully. If an applicant chooses not to utilize the health professions office and instead submits individual letters, some medical schools may not look favorably upon that decision especially if the health professions office/advisor at the college/university is well known for providing this service.

Each application service allows for a different number of letters to be submitted, so applicants should carefully review the application service requirements.

Application

Some of the application services require a photo of the applicant to be submitted as a component of the application. These photos should be conservative in nature. The applicant should be wearing appropriate clothing (not swimsuits, short dresses, or flaunting body parts) and be in an appropriate setting (not at a party). Cropping others out of a photo to display the applicant is also not advised. The best advice would be to have someone take a photo of him/her outside with a nice background wearing attire they might wear to the interview (detailed later in this chapter). The photo is not the time to show off some aspect of the applicant that is not appropriate for the professional setting.

*[handwritten margin note: * health professions packet contains letters from lots of ppl]*

Activities

The applications will require a listing of all activities since high school graduation. A lot of detail needs to be entered including: activity type, title, date range, hours per week, total hours, and a brief description of the activity. It is highly recommended that future applicants keep a log of all activities they are involved in from the point of graduating from high school

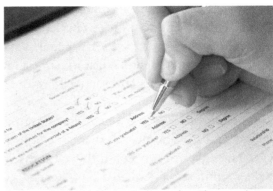

© jannoon028, 2014. Used under license from Shutterstock, Inc.

until (and after) the point of applying to medical school. It will make entering this information much easier. Often, applicants will not remember everything they have been involved in or the specifics of the activities. Additionally, applicants may feel that an activity that occurred several years ago is not as relative as one that is more recent, however the medical schools are looking at a longitudinal record so it may be important to include. Also, an applicant may think an activity that occurred only once (e.g., shadowing a physician for half a day) is not significant to include, however as part of the big picture that medical schools are considering, these activities may be important.

Keep a log of the following activities:

- health care exposure
- community service
- research
- leadership roles
- awards/honors
- extracurricular/leisure activities
- employment

AMCAS volunteering, leadership, allows a maximum of 15 activities (work, extracurricular, awards, honors, and/or publications) to be included, some of which will be designated as the most meaningful (https://www.aamc.org/students/applying/amcas/how_to_apply/129794/work_activities.html). TMDSAS does not have a cap on the number of activities an applicant can list, however applicants should be careful with how they list activities. Generally, schools are looking for quality over quantity. For example, an applicant does not need to list "Dean's List" four times for four different semesters. Those four semesters can be combined into one entry. This will be especially important for the AMCAS application given the cap of entries.

AMCAS also requires contact information to be listed to verify the activity so applicants should be careful to note this information as they keep their log of activities.

Health Care Exposure

While many people may have dreamed of becoming a physician since they were children, medical schools still want their motivation to be shown through their activities. Applicants should get involved in activities while in college (and after) that expose them to the field of medicine. In general, the expectation is that these experiences will help solidify that pursuing a career as a physician is what a student wants, and that it is based on a more realistic understanding of what the field entails.

Some people will have opportunities for health care exposure even in high school through specialized programs focused on health professions. Often these programs provide opportunities for not only coursework in health-related areas or in upper-level sciences, but also offer rotations in health professions as well as certifications such as Emergency Medical Technician or Certified Nursing Assistant. These are great early exposure experiences, however the TMDSAS application requires a listing of activities since graduating from high school. This is specifically written in the directions, so applicants *should not* enter activities completed in high school. Therefore, prospective applicants need to seek out first time or additional experiences once entering college. AMCAS and AACOMAS schools may also value more recent experiences completed in college, however these application services should be contacted to verify if high school entries are allowed to be included.

Shadowing

Some of the best direct experiences are through shadowing. Shadowing is when a volunteer observer follows a physician as they treat patients, make rounds, write medical notes, or perform surgery or other procedures. These experiences can occur in any setting from a domestic hospital, clinic, or at an international clinic or hospital. Some colleges/universities have organized programs with various hospitals and clinics that help coordinate these opportunities. Other times, these opportunities come about through approaching physicians directly.

Shadowing allows for direct observations of the physician's daily routine, of their interaction with patients, their treatment methods, bedside manner, interaction with other health care professionals, and behind-the-scenes duties as a physician. Often physicians will take the time to explain their methods or terminology to the person shadowing as well as provide or suggest reading resources on the cases they observed for additional learning. Just as with any experience involving others, professionalism is of the utmost importance in these opportunities. Students should be highly respectful of everyone involved and the sensitive nature of being allowed to interact with physicians while they work with patients.

Hospital Volunteering

Volunteering in a hospital is a common way to gain some exposure to medicine. Tasks can range greatly with little to no patient or physician interaction such as restocking supply closets and cleaning empty rooms to more interaction like visiting with patients or working with nurses or other health professions staff.

Some hospitals have a Child-Life program with a playroom for children who are patients and volunteers are able to play with the children. There are also pro-grams where volunteers can spend time with a patient such as an ill child while the parent(s) takes a break. Other hospitals have vol-unteer opportunities in the nurs-ery to rock newborn infants.

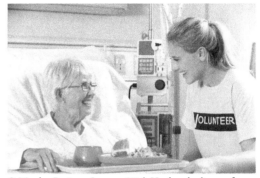

© MonkeyBusiness Images, 2014. Used under license from Shutterstock, Inc.

When seeking opportunities to volunteer at a hospital, students should inquire what tasks are available and if possible, choose the ones they are interested in. However, if a general opportunity exists to volunteer in the hospital, take it! It may not offer the chance to gain ex-posure to patients or physicians, but it could lead to those opportunities.

Health Career Employment

There are ways to work in the health care field even as a college student. Work-ing as a *scribe* is a great experience to obtain a wealth of exposure and knowl-edge in the hospital and clinic setting. Most scribe positions are offered through hospital emergency departments, however some individual clinics and physi-cians also have scribe positions. A scribe is an employee who works directly with the physician and records (either in writing or typing) the conversation between the physician and the patient, instructions from the physician to be noted in the patient's record, tests to be ordered, and any follow-up instruc-tions. These employees allow the physician to be free of the distraction of writ-ing notes as they interview the patient face-to-face knowing the conversation is being fully documented by the scribe.

Some students get direct employment experience by obtaining an Emer-gency Medical Technician license and working in various capacities. These employees can increase their skillset and advance into other positions such as a paramedic. Others work at various levels of nursing (which will require train-ing) or various medical technology positions.

Community Service

Getting into medical school is not just about grades and MCAT scores anymore. More and more medical schools are looking beyond academics for a well-rounded applicant who has been involved outside the class-room. Community service (non-health care related) is one of

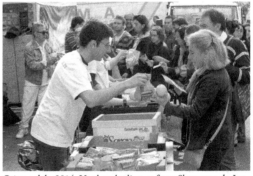

© imagelab, 2014. Used under license from Shutterstock, Inc.

those areas that medical schools may regard highly. Many medical schools are looking to admit applicants who have demonstrated compassion and a desire to serve others in meaningful ways and without compensation.

College students who are considering applying to medical school should get involved from their freshman year onward and volunteer not only on campus but off campus as well. There are many ways one can be involved. On-campus volunteering is the most feasible way for students to be involved. Volunteer opportunities are often required to be a member of certain student organizations. These may involve campus-wide cleanup events, fundraisers for various causes, or volunteering with community organizations.

Off-campus volunteering is also worthwhile and students or graduates can seek community volunteering on their own. Large organizations like Big Brothers Big Sisters of America, Habitat for Humanity, Best Buddies, and Special Olympics offer opportunities for volunteering. Other options include volunteering at a local nursing/retirement home, homeless shelter, and women's/children's shelter. Some students seek opportunities through Peace Corps or Teach For America, which have longer commitments.

Research

Undergraduate schools often offer opportunities to be involved in research, sometimes paid. If students are interested in research and would like to learn more about the scientific method and how to understand, interpret, and apply research methods and data, they should seek opportunities to be involved. These experiences do not need to be limited to basic science research. Some applicants may be interested in other areas such as psychology. There may also be summer clinical research opportunities at health care institutions.

Leadership

Future applicants should seek leadership opportunities through organizations or in the community. Leadership roles help develop communication and teamwork skills that will help in medical school. Physicians are regarded as leaders by the community, therefore developing these skills early will only help as they progress through their career.

Professionalism/Motivation/Honesty

Professionalism

Applicants should reflect that in pursuing a career as a physician, they will be interacting with many different people from advisors, faculty, classmates, patients, families, and health professions colleagues. Applicants need to recognize that positive, constructive interactions with others are important to the professional success as a physician. Social skills and appropriate interactions with others in various contexts, showing respect in communication, and ability to recognize what constitutes professional behavior are important for successful passage through this professional, highly regarded field.

When contacting medical schools via email, phone, or in person, applicants should always be respectful and courteous regardless of the role of the person they are speaking to. Interacting discourteously with members of an admissions office or pre-medical advising office will be considered behavioral/professional red flags. Prospective applicants should read medical school admissions' and application services' websites prior to inquiring with medical schools regarding questions that can be answered through those websites. Emails and phone calls regarding specific situations or to seek clarification are acceptable.

When contacting by phone, the applicant should speak confidently and respectfully, not be lethargic or unclear, and should also not interrupt during the conversation. When contacting through email, the applicant should not address with the informal greeting of "hey" or no name. The best approach is to use "Dr.", "Ms.", or "Mr." If an applicant utilizes social media, care should be taken when initiating a connection with those involved in the admissions process during this time. They should also be careful about sharing unprofessional comments, pictures, or activities on social media as they do not know the connection someone might have with the process.

DO-NOTs

Applicants should not call a medical school admissions office and demand to speak to "the person in charge." If an applicant feels his/her specific situation or questions would be best answered by the admissions office upper administration, the best approach is to ask if there is a process for doing so. The admissions office may allow for direct emails to be sent to admissions leaders or a phone or meeting appointment may be the protocol. Regardless, it is important to show respect for the communication process the office has established.

Applicants may interact with a variety of personnel during the application process. It is important to display the same level of respect and professionalism with all. Administrative Assistants should not be treated with disrespect or dismissed simply because an applicant does not deem them to have an impact in the decision-making process. Likewise, courteous interaction with medical students with whom the applicant may interact is also important. Applicants cannot assume the roles of individuals and the impact they have in the process. It is important to be sincere and genuine in all interactions. Applicants should not go into a medical school application process determined to impress or "butter-up" only those who they perceive to have a hand in the process. They should interact with all in a professional, genuine way.

Finally, medical school admissions administrators recognize that the application process is not only daunting; it is often stressful and overwhelming for applicants. Many applicants approach this process feeling it will determine the rest of their lives. Some have dreamed of becoming a physician for many years and they look at the admissions process as the last step to making their dreams a reality. With that in mind, sometimes the disappointment of the process reflects in poor decision-making regarding reaction and interaction with medical school admissions offices.

The following is an example of an inappropriate interaction with a medical school admissions office:

Carl has dreamed of becoming a physician since he was five years old. He has prepared his whole life for that moment. He is now a senior in college and has submitted all of his materials for his application to medical school. He was diligent in having his application complete and submitted early just as his pre-medical office had advised, but he's starting to get nervous because he has not heard back from the schools he has applied to. Several of his friends have been invited to interview and he knows their "stats" (MCAT and GPA) and wonders why he has not been invited since he thinks his stats are better. In a panicked moment, he decides to email each of the medical school admissions offices to inquire about his application. His first email is simply a request for the status of his application. When the response is that his file is "under review," it does nothing to ease his anxiety. They do not understand how big this is to him. He waits a few weeks and decides to email again, this time highlighting his many achievements. Maybe they are not aware of all he has accomplished (even though they have his application). After a few weeks of no response to this email, he is now angry. He sends another email stating that the medical school would be lucky to have a student like him and he knows he is better than several of the applicants the school has already interviewed. He receives no response.

What is wrong with this scenario? While the process to apply to medical school may be stressful and invoke anxiety when receiving no news or discouraging news, it is important the applicant remains professional. Medical schools receive all the documents they need to make their decision from the application services. They do not need applicants to relist everything they have accomplished. More importantly, emailing a medical school admissions office demanding to know why they have not been considered or coming across as entitled by making statements of perceived importance are quick ways to demonstrate unprofessionalism and/or possible instability.

Some things to remember:

1. Medical schools receive thousands of applications every year. There are many factors schools look for in determining which applicants are the right fit for them.
2. An applicant who compares him/herself to fellow applicants is missing the big picture. First, there is no way of knowing the full academic background of a fellow applicant, even if they share details. If a fellow applicant has low grades in his/her record, several withdrawals, or a low MCAT score, he/she may not share these details. Second, many medical schools are looking at more than just the academic record. Adding in the various life circumstances and experiences each applicant has makes them unique; therefore it is unreliable to compare them.
3. Professionalism includes autonomy from parents with the applicant acting as an independent adult in the process. Application documents are protected through the Family Educational Rights and Privacy Act (FERPA) making it unlawful for admissions personnel to discuss the application details with anyone other than the applicant. Parents and

significant others should not be enlisted to call admissions offices on the applicant's behalf.

Pre-Medical Advising Offices

When interacting with a pre-medical advising office at the undergraduate institution, an applicant should not be demanding in their requests and should be courteous and professional.

Here is an example of an inappropriate/unprofessional approach with a letter writer:

It is June of Sharron's junior year at her undergraduate institution. She plans to apply to medical school and realizes the application opened on May 1st. In the various workshops and handouts her pre-medical office has provided regarding the medical school application, as well as her own reading of the application service's website, she knows she will need two letters of recommendation from professors. She also remembers that despite the application deadline being several months away it is important to submit an early application to have the best chance of consideration. After a few days of enjoying her summer break, she decides to email her Biochemistry and Genetics professors to request a letter. Her emails are short and to the point asking that the letters be submitted within a week estimating that is how long it will take her to prepare her part of the application. One professor responds that he is away doing research at another institution and will need more time to write the letter. Sharron is upset that this professor does not realize how important this is to her and how quickly she needs to have the letters submitted. She emails him back stating just that. She thinks it is best to email the professor whom she has not heard from just in case he also does not realize and demand the letter be submitted by her one-week deadline.

What are the issues here? First, it is the applicant's responsibility to know the timeline of when the application is available, deadline dates, and the process for submitting letters. Second, it is courteous to provide letter writers at least one month's notice before the letters are due. Providing enough time to write the letter demonstrates respect and planning. Third, it is often helpful to set up an appointment and/or attach a résumé or curriculum vitae to the email so the letter writer is aware of all activities.

It may also be helpful to the letter writer to provide instructions on how to submit the letter and if a form must be attached. Some application services require that letters be uploaded by the letter writer into the system and be accompanied by a completed form signed by the applicant. Undergraduate schools that have a pre-medical office or a health professions advisory committee may have additional policies for submitting letters, such as interviewing with members of the committee before writing the letter. The applicant should research all of this before approaching letter writers, and do so months before the application opens.

Motivation

Motivation to become a physician is demonstrated through activities and education the student has pursued. Gaining health care exposure is not simply to understand more about the career, but also to show that it is the career choice the student wishes to pursue. Some applicants will have family members who are physicians and may have had opportunities to learn and observe the career through them. However, motivation to pursue medicine should be one's own demonstrated goal through their own involvement in health care experiences. It is not enough to say that one's mother or father is a physician, so outside experiences are not necessary. One's own activities is what demonstrates motivation.

Honesty

It should be obvious that honesty is an important characteristic that medical schools seek in applicants. It is *highly* important that applicants be entirely honest in their applications and interviews. While it may be enticing to leave out some unsatisfactory items like an academic conduct charge such as cheating or plagiarism or a criminal conviction, the applications asks for these items specifically and more and more medical schools run criminal background checks and drug tests on accepted students (see more under *Criminal Background* and *Academic Misconduct/Institutional Actions*).

Additionally, it is very important for the applicant to use their original work in all of their essays. These essays should be personal and unique, however there are people and companies who provide fully or partially written essays for purchase. Applicants should refrain from using such essays. They should also be careful when asking others to edit their essay, which results in an essay that is no longer the applicant's own due to extensive feedback by the reviewer. Finally, it may be tempting to embellish or make up health care experiences, community service, awards, leadership, etc., and include them under the activity listing; however, the applicant will likely be asked to discuss these events further and if it seems the applicant cannot talk much about these experiences or has embellished, it could be enough to deter the interviewer from recommending for admission.

Personal Statement

The personal statement is an applicant's opportunity to provide a narrative describing the motivation to pursue medicine as well as give some insight into his/her personality. All other parts of the application are descriptions or listings of what an applicant has accomplished or been involved in. However, the personal statement is where an admissions administrator and/or committee member can get to know an applicant even better.

For the personal statement, applicants will write about their motivation for medicine. This may seem an easy task, however an applicant should spend some time thinking about his/her motivation, how it has been developed, and what experiences he/she has had to support it. The essays include a character/word count limit, so the applicant will need to be concise and effective in their message. For many applicants, it is difficult to put into words why they want to be a doctor beyond the general notions of wanting to help others and enjoying their science background. However, a well-written personal statement is one that provides a more in-depth description of one's desire to pursue this career, and many admissions committee members place heavy weight on this statement. Grammatical and spelling errors should also be avoided.

The TMDSAS application includes one additional required essay and one optional essay. Applicants are encouraged to share more about themselves by utilizing these essays. Care should be taken not to repeat what was already written and instead expand upon an experience alluded to in the personal statement or share something new not covered elsewhere. Additional essay may be required as part of the secondary applications.

Criminal Convictions and Academic Misconduct

The applications will contain a section on criminal background and academic misconduct/institutional action. Just as with the rest of the application, it is very important that an applicant honestly and fully answer these questions. The information is often verified and if any discrepancies exist or dishonesty is found, an application may be rejected or if an offer of admission has been made, the offer could be rescinded.

Criminal Background

If an applicant has received a misdemeanor or felony charge that is currently on his/her record, they should respond honestly to that portion of the application. More and more medical schools are conducting criminal background checks on accepted applicants. If the applicant failed to indicate the charge on the application, yet it is reported on the criminal background check, the applicant places himself/herself in the position of possibly having the offer of acceptance rescinded due to the discrepancy. In the applications there is an opportunity to explain what the details of the incident were. Applicants should read the TMDSAS, AMCAS, and AACOMAS websites thoroughly for detailed information on what to report in this section.

Applicants should also realize that many state medical licensing boards will also do criminal background checks and physicians waiting to be approved to practice medicine in that state may have to go before the board to explain their record. Additionally, more and more hospitals where third and fourth year medical students are doing rotations are requesting their own criminal background checks as well as drug tests.

Academic Misconduct/Institutional Actions

If an applicant has received a charge of academic misconduct such as cheating, plagiarism, or other institutional violations it is important to honestly answer this question as well. Often these charges are found on an applicant's transcript; therefore the applicant does not want any discrepancies to arise.

For both these situations, it is important that the applicant not only disclose any incidents but also provide a description of what occurred and what they have learned from it. Again, applicants need to read each application service's website to verify what needs to be included.

Undergraduate Majors

Many medical schools do not have a preference for the applicant's undergraduate major. The majority of applicants major in the basic sciences (biology, chemistry, physics, etc.), however applicants who major in other disciplines are considered for admission as well. Typically applicants are encouraged to pursue the major that most interests them, keeping in mind that if it is a nonscience major, the prerequisite courses will need to planned in.

Pre-Requisite Courses

If an applicant chooses a major outside of the sciences, it will be important they review the pre-requisite course requirements for the medical schools they will be applying to as many of these will be science courses. It would be helpful for these students to also consider taking additional upper-level science courses to better prepare for the first year of medical school.

Students should also review the sections of the MCAT to ensure they have the academic background necessary to do well. More information on the MCAT can be found in the *MCAT/GPA* section later in this chapter and in *Chapter 2: The Undergraduate Premedical Coursework and Requirements.*

Community College Coursework

When students are attending a four-year institution from which they will earn their degree, they should aim to complete all of their science coursework from that institution, whenever possible. An applicant who has taken all or the majority of their science pre-requisites from community colleges during the summer breaks while at home, for example, raises a red flag for many medical schools.

There are some instances when applicants will have community college credit on their transcript. More and more high school students are taking dual-credit courses allowing them the opportunity to earn college credit. Others will begin their college career at a community college before transferring to a four-year institution. These scenarios are acceptable, however applicants are encouraged to take additional upper-level science courses at their four-year institution.

MCAT/GPA

A helpful resource for applicants to locate each medical school's entering class data such as MCAT and GPA is the Medical School Admissions Requirements

(MSAR) produced by the AAMC. This tool can also allow the applicant to read mission statements, learn about deadline dates, medical school class profiles, and cost of attendance. More information can be found at: https://www.aamc.org/students/applying/requirements/msar/.

MCAT

The MCAT is required to be considered for admission into medical school. In the spring of 2015, a new version of the MCAT was released. This exam includes the following sections:

- Critical Analysis and Reasoning Skills
- Biological and Biochemical Foundations of Living Systems
- Chemical and Physical Foundations of Biological Systems
- Psychological, Social, and Biological Foundations of Behavior

The exam is computer-based and is offered several times a year from January through September. More information on the MCAT can be found at: https://www.aamc.org/students/applying/mcat/. The MCAT is also covered in *Chapter 2: The Undergraduate Premedical Coursework and Requirements.*

A good score on the MCAT is important to demonstrate the ability to do well on standardized exams. What is a "good score"? Most schools will publish their recent matriculated class's MCAT average. That will give the applicant a good indication of what score to aim for to be competitive for the schools he/she will be applying to. Of course, averages mean that there is a range, however the closer to the average or above will help the applicant be more competitive. The subsection scores are also important.

Medical schools have varying policies on whether they give weight to the highest score or most recent score. All scores will be reported to the application services and medical school interview screeners and admissions committees will see every score. For this reason, it is highly discouraged for applicants to take the MCAT before they have taken the necessary pre-requisite courses, are adequately prepared, or do so just to get an idea on where they will score as a baseline. Each score will be part of the permanent record once released. TMDSAS schools consider MCAT scores not older than five years. Most AMCAS schools require that scores are no more than three years old. Because there are differences, applicants should review each medical school's website for the MCAT policy.

MCAT scores are considered by many schools to be part of a complete application. If an applicant chooses to take the MCAT during the application window (when the application is available through to the deadline date), scores are not released for approximately one month following the test date. If the applicant has submitted every other required document but is waiting on an MCAT score, medical schools will often not review the application until the score has been received. This is also often the case for a repeat MCAT score, even if the previous score was competitive.

Applicants should also review the Fee Assistant Program (FAP) through the AAMC to determine if they qualify for a discount on the cost of the

MCAT. More information can be found at: https://www.aamc.org/students /applying/fap/.

Grade Point Average (GPA)

The GPA is an important academic record and informs admissions committees not only of the applicant's academic preparedness but also grade trends and readiness for the medical school curriculum, especially the first two years (see *Chapter 7: Medical School Curriculum Preclinical Years*).

TMDSAS calculates the overall GPA using every course the applicant has received college credit for, including graduate courses and dual credit courses taken in high school. So even when an applicant has retaken a course or taken courses at various institutions, all grades will still be calculated into the overall GPA. TMDSAS also does not factor in "+" or "−" grades as an institution might. AMCAS calculates the GPA using every course with semester (or quarter) hours and a letter grade. AMCAS converts applicants' transcript grades to AMCAS grades for standardization. This conversion gives weight to +/− grades. More information can be found here: https://students-residents .aamc.org/applying-medical-school/article/section-4-course-work/. AACOMAS does assign a numerical value to +/− grades in calculating the GPA.

The GPA may be reported to medical schools through the application in many different ways. Reports may provide an overall GPA, undergraduate science (Biology, Chemistry, Physics, Math-BCPM-GPA) and non-science GPA, and graduate overall, science, and non-science GPA. GPAs will also be broken down by year (e.g., freshman through senior, post-baccalaureate, and graduate). This provides the medical schools with the opportunity to see what improvements the applicant has made over time or to balance a lower overall GPA with a higher post-baccalaureate science GPA.

It is very important for future applicants to work hard to maintain a strong GPA. After a student has earned a number of credits, it becomes more and more difficult to increase their overall GPA. While medical schools may look at grade trends and individual course grades when an overall GPA is lower, there are thousands of applicants applying to medical schools each year, therefore, the stronger the GPA throughout, the more chances to be considered for an interview. Grades in science courses (particularly upper-level courses) are especially important as they are the most in-line with what will be studied during the first year of medical school. Options for improving a GPA through postbaccalaureate work are described in *Chapter 4: Nontraditional/ Veteran/Military Applicants*.

Dual Degree Options

Some medical schools offer dual degree options in combination with the MD (Doctor of Medicine) or DO (Doctor of Osteopathic Medicine) and require the applicant to indicate their intent to apply on the application. Programs may include a dual degree with another terminal degree such as a PhD (Doctor of Philosophy) or JD (Juris Doctor), while others offer them with master-level graduate degrees such as MPH (Master of Public Health), MBA (Master of Business Administration), and MS (Master of Science). Some schools will ask your intention to apply to the master-level programs on the application, while others will not.

Dual degrees will require varied additional years to medical school (i.e., 1–5 years). Applicants should review these possibilities before applying so they are prepared to apply to those programs as well. More details on dual degrees are covered in *Chapter 6: Joint Degree Medical Programs*.

Application Submission Timing

The applications open in May of every year. Deadline dates may vary and may seem to the applicant to be far in the future allowing plenty of time to complete the application, however it is still important for an applicant to submit early in the process. For TMDSAS medical schools, the deadline is October 1st, however, it is recommended that an applicant complete and submit their application and all supporting and required documents (including secondary applications) before or during the summer months. Many TMDSAS medical schools begin interviews in early August (some even in late July); therefore they are screening applications in June and July to fill those interview slots. For AMCAS and AACOMAS schools, interviewing may occur into the spring semester, however early application submission may still be recommended.

As addressed above under the "MCAT/GPA" section, a pending MCAT score will often keep the applicant's file from being reviewed even if the rest of the application is complete including a previous MCAT score.

Holistic Admissions

More and more medical schools are reviewing the application as a whole rather than just metrics or other very specific aspects to grant interviews. Each medical school considers different aspects as a fit for the mission of their medical school. For example, some medical schools are heavily focused on research and highly value an applicant's research activities while others may be committed to producing primary care physicians and therefore look for similar activities in the applicant's record.

A holistic approach allows a medical school to look beyond metrics (MCAT and GPA) and consider the experiences and traits that are important to meet their mission. This may mean they regard medical exposure and community service just as highly as academics. An applicant's background such as overcoming hardship or adversity, experiences, or the exhibition of certain traits such as compassion or altruism may also be regarded highly by a medical school.

The AAMC has developed an official pathway for medical schools to implement a holistic review process in their admissions selection. More information can be found on the Holistic Review Project at the following site: https://www.aamc.org/initiatives/holisticreview/.

Interview

The interview is a necessary part of the process for gaining admission to medical school. Schools will review the full application and make a decision to invite an applicant for an in-person interview at the medical school. This interview (followed by the admissions committee meeting) is typically the last step for determining acceptability for a program.

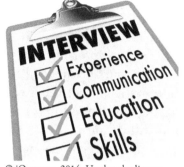

© iQoncept, 2014. Used under license from Shutterstock, Inc.

Schools use many and often different variables to determine admission to their program. Often, they are looking for characteristics and/or a record of accomplishments or participation in activities that fit their mission and the kind of physician they want to train (as described previously under *Holistic Admissions*).

The interview day is composed of many activities to help an applicant get acquainted with the school, students, faculty, and facilities. Some schools may even have a two-day interview schedule. Regardless, applicants should be prepared for a full day of activities and therefore should plan on getting good sleep the evening before.

The Invitation

Schools will most likely contact applicants via phone or email to invite for the interview. Some may invite on a specific date not giving the applicant a choice. Others will provide an option to either select the date provided or request an alternate date. If there is a conflict with the day they have provided, it may be helpful to contact the school via phone to ask if there is a possibility to reschedule. The key here is to be courteous and respectful and certainly not demand that the request be granted. They may or may not be able to accommodate the change and expecting that the change be granted is not the correct approach. Most medical schools interview during the work week, therefore applicants should be prepared to ask professors to make up work in missed classes or ask a supervisor for a day off work.

Applicants should be very careful to read the information received about the interview thoroughly. Often the invitation will include directions and maps to the location, parking information, time of arrival, and an outline of the day. More information will likely be provided upon arrival so applicants should not be surprised if they have the bare minimum information beforehand. For example, many schools will not provide in advance the actual time of the interviews or with whom the applicant will be interviewing.

The information will likely also provide instructions on how to respond to the invitation. This is very important. If the school requests a confirmation of the interview date and/or time, it is imperative to follow through with this request as soon as possible or there is a risk the spot will be given to another applicant. Since much of the communication with the medical school will be via email, applicants should regularly check their SPAM folder throughout the interview season, as bulk emails are often filtered as SPAM.

Interview Day Activities

Each medical school will have their own unique schedule of activities for the day, however beyond the actual interviews, activities will most likely include tours of the facilities, a student panel, and a presentation covering information about the medical school. The interviews will be at some point during the day, sometimes in the morning, sometimes in the afternoon, sometimes both.

The interview day may be an overwhelming experience with so much information to absorb, meeting other candidates, and the possible feeling of intimidation at interviewing with medical school faculty. Applicants should try to familiarize themselves with the school before getting there (actually, this should have been done when applying). This will help reduce anxiety. Materials like medical school brochures and other informational documents will likely be provided, however it is a good idea to bring a pen and small notebook for taking notes throughout the day.

Applicants should also write down their gut-feeling perceptions of the day. They should include the aspects they liked and did not like and their overall feeling of the environment, facilities, students, resources, curriculum, etc. If an applicant is interviewing at more than one medical school and several months pass before they have to make a decision, these notes will be helpful to recall what the initial impression of the school was. It is important to use the interview day experience to help determine if the applicant feels it would be a good fit for him/her. Not all applicants will have the freedom to choose between multiple offers from medical schools in which case they will be happy if they receive any offer of acceptance. However, in the case of multiple offers, assessing which program is the right fit will be an important decision. Before the interview, applicants should write down questions they would like to ask the faculty/administrators/students they meet. The interview day is the time to get those answered.

It is appropriate to send "thank you" cards to interviewers following the interview day, however they should not be pre-written and brought to the interview to be handed out immediately following the interview as this comes across as disingenuous.

The Handshake

While it may seem like it would not make a big impact, a solid handshake is important when meeting new people, especially in a professional interview setting. Applicants should expect to shake hands with many people on interview day including interviewers. The handshake should not be overpowering, however it should also not be limp. A solid, firm grip should be used. People can form opinions based on this interaction alone, including assuming the lack of confidence or disinterest (when a limp or loose handshake is used) or overconfidence, aggressive (if an overpowering handshake is used). Applicants can easily practice this with others.

If an applicant has religious or other reasons/obligations for being unable to shake hands of certain people, he/she should practice explaining succinctly why this is so as they will most likely be faced with having to do so on an interview day.

Interview Format

Medical schools may interview in different formats and may utilize people in various roles to interview.

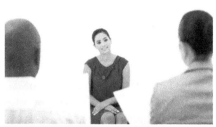

© michaeljung, 2014. Used under license from Shutterstock, Inc.

- Panel Interview: This would consist of more than one interviewer at the same time.
- One-on-One Interview: This is the most common type of interview and include only the applicant and the interviewer.
- Multiple Mini-Interview (MMI): This process uses short sessions (sometimes 5–8 minutes each) in a timed circuit of about 6–10 stations. Each station will involve something different from a standard interview question, working through an ethical scenario,

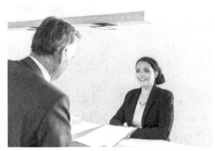

© Frank Gaertner, 2014. Used under license from Shutterstock, Inc.

interacting with an actor, or completing a task. Faculty at McMaster University in Canada developed this format. (Eva, K. W., H. I. Reiter, J. Rosenfeld, G. R. Norman. 2004. "An Admissions OSCE: The Multiple Mini-interview." *Medical Education* 2004, 38:314–326.)

Just as there are different types of interviews, there are also different types of information the interviewers are provided. Some interviewers are fully informed about the applicant, while others may go into the interview blind. Thus, it is important not to make assumptions about what aspects of the application the interviewer has had access to.

- Closed-File Interview: This typically refers to an interviewer having only the biographical information from an application to review for the interview. This may include the activities, awards, honors, and personal statements, but not the academic information (GPA and/or MCAT and academic record).
- Blind Interview: A blind interview typically means the interviewer has no information about the applicant or very little such as undergraduate institution.
- Open-File Interview: Interviewers will likely have all or most parts of the application, including activities, personal statements, and academic information but in some cases not letters of recommendation.

Most interviews will be 30 minutes long, but there may be some variation to this, especially if a panel interview or MMI are used.

Schools utilize people in various roles to interview candidates. Some interviewers may be PhD or MD/DO faculty members, community physicians, administrators in leadership roles, and/or medical students. No interviewer should ever be taken lightly by the applicant. For example, an applicant may feel they could relax with a medical student interviewer, however they should be mindful that students might have a highly respected voice or even vote on the admissions committee. Each interview may be completely different. There is often no way to predict what an interviewer will ask, although there are some topics an applicant can prepare for (described below under *Practice–Mock Interviews*). Applicants can practice their skills in mock interviews with faculty members or mentors. Most medical schools utilize a uniform evaluation instrument so they may be attempting to cover certain areas in the interview to help them evaluate the applicant based on what the admissions committee is looking for.

Professional Attire

The interview day is a professional event and the applicant needs to look the part. Medical school is a professional environment (similar to law school and other graduate-level programs), which is different from most undergraduate schools. Applicants should be prepared to dress professionally (i.e., suit). This may be the first time the applicant has ever worn a suit and if so, he/she should request help from someone who may have knowledge of which suits would look best on the applicant. Many applicants choose to wear black suits, however other shades are appropriate as well such as dark grey/charcoal or navy.

Female applicants should consider the following when selecting their interview day attire:

- Pantsuits (a suit that has two separate but matching pieces—slacks and a suit jacket) or skirt suits are both appropriate. Often this will depend on what she is comfortable wearing.
- The suit should fit well, but not be too tight. The blouse worn underneath the suit jacket should not be low-cut or have a deep plunge showing cleavage.
- The pants or skirt should also not be too tight. The skirt should not be too short; the applicant should not need to tug at the skirt throughout the interview. A highly suggested length of the skirt is no shorter than an inch above the knees.
- The shoes should be comfortable. If a heel is chosen, she should have practiced walking in them and be prepared to walk around the medical school campus for tours. Traditionally, a closed-toe shoe is recommended rather than open-toe. It is appropriate to bring more comfortable shoes for the tours however these should be professional as well.
- Hair and make-up should be appropriate and not overdone.

Male applicants should consider the following when selecting an interview day suit:

- Enlist the assistance of a salesperson or friend/family member who has experience selecting suits to ensure the right fit. Often applicants who have never worn suits before select a size that is too big leaving the shoulders too broad for the body.

- The button-up dress shirt worn underneath the suit jacket should compliment the color of the suit and not be too bright.
- A tie should be worn with the colors complimenting the shirt and suit and again not be too bright in color.
- The shoes should be polished. Appropriately colored dress socks should be worn (not white gym socks).

It should be an obvious point, however applicants should never wear tennis shoes or casual shoes such as flip-flops to the interview. Shoes should also be scuff free and clean. Jeans or t-shirts should also not be worn. It is always a safe bet to wear a suit unless the medical school recommends something different. Applicants should also practice good hygiene, especially on interview day, showering the morning of the interview, brushing teeth, and fixing hair appropriately, wear deodorant, as well as taking care to clean under fingernails. If female applicants have nail polish on, the polish should not be chipped. All of these subtleties may make an impression and the applicant does not want that to be a negative impression simply based on appearance.

Here are some good and bad examples of interview attire:

Females: **Males:**

| Good | Bad | Good | Bad |

© Viorel Sima, 2014. Used under license from Shutterstock, Inc.
© Minerva Studio, 2014. Used under license from Shutterstock, Inc.
© pzAxe, 2014. Used under license from Shutterstock, Inc.
© Odua Images, 2014. Used under license from Shutterstock, Inc.
© originalpunkt, 2014. Used under license from Shutterstock, Inc.

Practice – Mock Interviews

While it is impossible to predict what and how many questions an interviewer will ask, there are still general ways an applicant can prepare for the interview. It would be helpful to find a professor, professional, or friend who has some experience to provide feedback on the applicant's communication skills as well as answer-quality. Some undergraduate pre-medical advising offices offer the opportunity to participate in mock-interviews and if so, the applicant should take advantage of them. If not, there are some general ways to prepare.

One question that an applicant should be prepared to answer is his/her motivation for becoming a physician. This seems like the most obvious question one should be able to answer, especially since it is written about in the personal statement, however it is often one of the more difficult answers to articulate verbally. Applicants should not plan to have pat or rehearsed answers to questions as that will likely come across to the interviewer as disingenuous, therefore the applicant should feel comfortable talking through their experiences and motivation. Applicants should read about and understand current health and social issues and topics and be able to communicate about them.

Nerves

It is normal for applicants to be nervous on interview day. Admissions personnel recognize this and usually do what they can to ease nerves. However, the day will be full of activities and meeting many new people. It is helpful for applicants to be aware of what makes them nervous and how they cope with those feelings.

Sometimes the result of nerves is talking too much, too fast, too loudly, too softly, or not talking at all. While for others it means sweating excessively, stammering, laughing uncontrollably, crying, or even becoming physically ill. Whatever symptoms the applicant may feel, he/she should have a good grasp on coping with and overcoming these feelings. Going through mock interviews is a good way to put oneself in an uncomfortable position during which they will have to talk about their goals, motivation for medicine, describe their activities, and talk through how they might handle an ethical scenario. An applicant does not want this to be the reason they were unable to convey their motivation for medicine accurately or to misrepresent who they are.

It is generally not seen in a positive light if an applicant asks for feedback immediately following the interview. Applicants should refrain from asking, "How did I do?" as it may reflect insecurity or immaturity.

Communicating with Admissions Offices

The first part of communicating with admissions offices is providing all the information requested on the application. This may not require communicating directly with the office, however if information should change, such as contact information, the applicant should follow the correct protocol for notifying either the application service or the schools directly.

The next time an applicant is likely to correspond with an admissions office is when invited for an interview. Often an interview invitation comes with a required response. The medical school may call the applicant to offer the interview invitation or they may send an email. Regardless of the method used, the applicant should pay close attention to the directions provided as the invitation often requires a reply. It is important to be timely with the reply or risk losing the interview invitation. These details also apply if an offer of acceptance is made.

Canceling/Rescheduling an Interview

If an applicant must cancel or reschedule an interview, it is important and courteous to try to provide the most notice possible. Sometimes last minute emergencies arise leaving the applicant with no choice but to cancel or ask to reschedule the day before or of an interview. Outside of these scenarios, the applicant should provide as much notice as possible (preferably two weeks or more). Contact should be made by both calling the admissions office and sending an email. If the applicant wishes to reschedule an interview, he/she should ask if it is allowable and explain the reason for the request, but not expect it to be accommodated.

If an applicant has changed his/her mind about interviewing at a particular medical school and has already confirmed an interview date, professional courtesy is to contact the school two weeks or more before the scheduled interview and request to cancel (and withdraw the application). Under no circumstances should the applicant not notify the school and simply not show up for the interview. There are great resources and coordination required for interview day including time taken off by faculty members and administrators to interview, so a lack of notification is inexcusable, inconsiderate, and unprofessional.

Selection Process

The selection process varies slightly from one application service to another. Below each of the processes will be highlighted.

TMDSAS

The Texas process tends to occur earlier than the rest of the nation. Texas medical schools that utilize TMDSAS (currently the only medical school in Texas that does not is Baylor College of Medicine, the only private medical school in Texas) begin interviewing in early August (some may begin a bit earlier, some a bit later). Interviews typically take place weekly and proceed until either mid-December or early January.

Pre-Match

Texas residents who interviewed at a TMDSAS school(s) are eligible to receive pre-match offers between November 15th and December 31st. Applicants may receive multiple pre-match offers and have the option of accepting all of the offers during this period of time.

Match

Approximately mid-January, any applicant who interviewed at one or more TMDSAS medical school(s) (whether they received an offer or not during the pre-match period), would submit a rank list of those schools via the TMDSAS portal. This is in preparation for the match process that occurs on or around February 1st, which matches the applicant to a medical school based on the applicant's preferences and the medical schools' rank lists. The match process serves to fill any remaining seats each of the medical schools have following the pre-match process. More information about the pre-match and match process can be found at: http://www.tmdsas.com/medical/acceptance_Match_info.html#PreMatchOffers.

Here is an example of an applicant's ranking decisions:

- Applicant James applies to all TMDSAS medical schools. He is fortunate enough to receive five interviews in the fall. Since he submitted his application in late June, he interviewed at the five schools between August and October. On November 15th, he checks his email and has two new emails from schools where he interviewed offering him a seat in their class (Schools A and B). With their offer, they provide him two weeks to make a decision. He is torn because he can see himself attending both schools and feels he needs more information and time to decide. He remembers that he is allowed to accept both offers during the pre-match period (November 15–December 31), so he responds immediately to both accepting their offers and provides the requested paperwork holding his spot at those two schools.

- A week later, he is pleasantly surprised to find an email with a third offer of admission to another TMDSAS school (School C). Once again, he can see himself attending this school so he responds that he would like to accept the offer. With the three pre-match offers, he realizes that one of the first two schools would likely not be on his top choice. Therefore, he decides to notify School A via email immediately. He sends a courteous email thanking School A for their offer but due to other offers he has received, he would like to decline the offer and withdraw his application.

- Now James is holding a seat at Schools B and C. December 31st comes and goes and he does not receive pre-match offers from Schools D and E. He checks TMDSAS for the January deadline by which he must submit his match rankings. He could choose to rank one of his pre-match offers as #1, which would eliminate the rest of the schools. However, he weighs his options and decides to rank as follows:

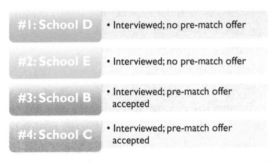

#1: School D	• Interviewed; no pre-match offer
#2: School E	• Interviewed; no pre-match offer
#3: School B	• Interviewed; pre-match offer accepted
#4: School C	• Interviewed; pre-match offer accepted

In this scenario, he would not put his seat at Schools B or C in jeopardy because he ranked them #3 and #4. Through the match process, if he does not match to either School D or E, he would match to School B. School C's seat would no longer be available to him since he ranked School B higher.

*He does not rank School A since he decided to decline their offer and withdraw his application during the pre-match period.

In the meantime, the medical schools are also submitting their rank lists of applicants they interviewed to TMDSAS. In February, the match will occur and James logs into his TMDSAS portal to learn the outcome, which is as follows:

Scenario 1:

In Scenario 1, James has matched to #3 School B, one of the schools he received a pre-match offer from.

- He will likely be on the alternate list at #1 School D and #2 School E.
- #4 School C's offer goes away because he matched to a higher-ranked school. He no longer has this school as an option.

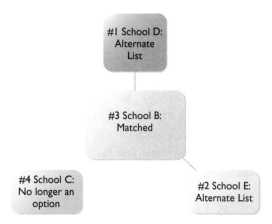

Scenario 2:

In Scenario 2, James matched to #2 School E, one of the schools he did not receive a pre-match offer from.

- He will likely be on the alternate list at #1 School D.
- #3 School B and #4 School C are no longer options since he matched to a higher-ranked school.

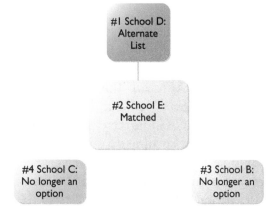

James could have also have matched to his #1 ranked school in which case the remaining schools' offers would no longer be available since he matched to his highest-ranked school.

Ultimately, applicants are encouraged to rank by preference of attendance regardless of pre-match offers, no offers, or a mixed scenario. Here is another scenario James could have chosen:

#1: School B	• Interviewed; pre-match offer accepted
#2: School E	• Interviewed; no pre-match offer
#3: School C	• Interviewed; pre-match offer accepted
#4: School D	• Interviewed; no pre-match offer

In this scenario, he ranks one of his pre-match offers #1. This would eliminate all other schools since he has chosen a pre-match offer as his most preferred school, including those he did not receive a pre-match offer from.

Alternate/Waitlist

If an applicant has a seat at a TMDSAS medical school through this process and is on another school(s) alternate list (such as in Scenarios 1 and 2 above), the potential exists to be made an offer for a seat from the alternate list until the close of business on June 1st. After June 1st, TMDSAS medical schools can no longer make offers to applicants holding a seat at another TMDSAS medical school. The dates for non-Texas residents and non-TMDSAS medical schools are different and described below.

Non-Texas Residents

If an applicant is a non-Texas resident applying through the TMDSAS process, they do not go through the pre-match or match process described above. TMDSAS medical schools can begin making offers to non-Texas residents on October 15th and can make rolling offers after that until matriculation. TMDSAS medical schools (all Texas public medical schools) are state-mandated to accept 90% Texas residents.

Special Programs

The TMDSAS medical schools have a number of special program with differing deadline dates. More information about the programs and requirements and deadline dates can be found at http://www.tmdsas.com/medical/special-programs.html

AMCAS

Most MD granting medical schools in the United States (including Puerto Rico) utilize AMCAS. This includes the only private medical school in Texas, Baylor College of Medicine. There is no systematic pre-match or match process through AMCAS like there is in TMDSAS. Aside from the main policies such as application opening date and dates which applicants need to narrow down multiple offers to one, each medical school within AMCAS designates their own deadline. Typically, these schools will interview throughout the application period. Many interview in both the fall and spring semesters and make offers of admissions during that time on a rolling basis.

A list of AMCAS participating medical schools can be found here: https://www.aamc.org/students/applying/amcas/participating_schools/

Holding Multiple Offers

Applicants who are holding multiple seats to AMCAS schools along with a TMDSAS school following match can hold those seats until April 30th. Applicants should notify all schools from which they wish to withdraw based on this date and hold only one seat after that time.

AACOMAS

All DO granting medical schools in the United States, except the University of North Texas Health Science Center Texas College of Osteopathic Medicine, which utilizes TMDSAS, utilize AACOMAS. Similar to the AMCAS schools, AACOMAS schools may interview in both the fall and spring semesters and make rolling offers during that time. Applicants should look at each school's website to determine deadline dates, many of which have a February 1st deadline, although some may be before or after.

Gap Year(s)

A gap year is a year following graduation from undergraduate school when the applicant has not matriculated into medical school. Sometimes this is planned while other times it occurs due to not being accepted into medical school on the first application.

A gap year is not necessarily regarded negatively by medical schools. Even though the traditional applicant is applying just before and during their senior year of college, many other applicants apply after graduating or even after having another career discussed more in *Chapter 4: Nontraditional/Veteran/Military Applicants.*

In order for a gap year to be viewed positively, it should be used in a productive way. Applicants should plan for employment, preferably in a field applicable to their future careers in medicine. This can be through research, medical-related work, service industry where they are caring for others, etc. If they are unable to gain work in such fields, they should plan to stay involved in gaining health care experience and volunteering in the community. Other people will have opportunities for extensive volunteering or overseas experiences. Still others may use the time to take additional coursework or earn an advanced degree to better prepare for medical school or dedicate time to studying for the MCAT.

There is no one perfect timeline for getting into medical school. Admissions Committees know there are various circumstances and reasons why applicants have different pathways.

Reapplication

Since the process for gaining admission into medical school is highly competitive, many applicants find themselves in a position to have to reapply. If an applicant is not successful in gaining admission, he/she should schedule an appointment with his/her pre-medical advisor to talk through their application and request feedback. Contacting the medical schools he/she applied to is also appropriate. Some medical schools offer the opportunity for a "file review," which is feedback regarding the application and suggestions for improvements upon a reapplication. This should be requested after the interview season has ended. In Texas, that would be mid-January. For AMCAS schools, it would be best to contact the school for the best time to request a file review (if provided).

The TMDSAS application asks whether the applicant has previously applied to medical school and to which schools. It also provides the applicant space to indicate what they have done since last applying. This is a great opportunity for the applicant to highlight the key things they have done to improve. AMCAS and AACOMAS may not provide the opportunity to explain, however there should be evidence the applicant has continued to improve over the year.

A reapplication is not typically seen as a red flag to medial schools unless the applicant did nothing to improve from the previous application. If improvement was made, especially significant improvement, reapplications often show motivation and dedication to pursuing the goal of becoming a physician.

Key areas to consider:

- MCAT score – Is there a need to increase the score? Medical schools will typically disclose their most recently matriculated average MCAT score. This will give the applicant an idea of what to aim for.
- GPA – This is typically not an area that is easily remedied in a year's time between applications. Sometimes the applicant may need to complete pre-requisite courses or take additional courses to show a continued upward-trend in grades. Other times the applicant needs to plan for significant ways to improve the academic record to show admissions committees his/her preparedness for medical school (see *Post-Baccalaureate and Graduate Degrees* section in Chapter 4).
- Health care exposure – Often this is the area where medical schools can provide some insight, however applicants can generally ascertain whether they have had quality experiences and enough health care exposure. Did the exposure provide contact with physicians and/or patients? Did the experience only allow for minimal exposure such as hospital volunteer time spent restocking linens? Was there enough variety? Has the exposure been over a period of at least a year or was the time spent only within months of the application? Has the last experience been several years in the past?
- Community service – Applicants should spend some time volunteering in the community (non-health care related). If the previous application contained a record of very little to no community service, the applicant should spend time doing so before reapplying.
- Research – Research exposure will not be on the radar of all medical schools, which is why it is important for applicants to look into what each school values. If the applicant is particularly interested in medical schools that value a record of research exposure, it will be important to seek out opportunities in this area. For other medical schools, research experience is not necessary to be competitive.
- Timing of the application – Even though the applications provide several months from the open of the application to the deadline, it is in the best interest of the applicant to apply early in the application season. If the previous application was submitted later in the season, closer to the deadline date(s), the plan should be to complete and submit the reapplication much earlier. Keep in mind this may also include an MCAT retest. If a retest is planned during the application window, scores are not released for approximately one month following the test date and medical schools will often not review applications until the new score has been received.

- Essays – Sometimes a personal statement describing one's motivation for medicine does not do the applicant's passion and motivation justice. There are varied opinions on what makes a personal statement good, therefore it is often difficult to get the same advice, however an applicant can still read through their essays and decide whether they conveyed their motivation thoroughly, provided examples and details of experiences they have had, and have given the reader a glimpse into their personality.

- Interview skills (communication) – Most medical schools will not give the applicant feedback about the previous interviews, however applicants with good insight can reflect back to the interviews and think about the following: did they express themselves thoroughly without going overboard?; did they stay on track with the questions or were they tangential in their responses?; did their nerves impact them negatively causing them to talk too much, too little, seem incongruent (laugh while discussing a serious experience or observation)?; did they get stuck on some of the questions finding themselves unable to provide answers?; and/or did they provide answers which showed depth rather than superficial knowledge on topics like current issues, ethical dilemmas, and/or the field of medicine?

- Letters of recommendation – Applicants traditionally wave their right to view letters of recommendation (which is recommended by most medical schools), however applicants can think about whether they chose individuals who may not have known them well or the applicant may not have adequately informed them about their background, motivation, and activities. It is recommended that applicants not ask for previous year's letters to be forwarded to be used with a reapplication. The applicant should instead reconnect (or preferably, maintain contact) with their original letter writers, updating them on their new experiences and renewed motivation. They can also seek out new letter writers based on activities from their recent experiences.

These are just some reasons why an applicant may not have been considered during the interview process, however it is through the feedback from an informed source that will be the most beneficial in determining how to proceed on a reapplication.

The application process can be daunting and overwhelming, but each school and application service provides information and data to help inform applicants about the process as well as what is most important. It is up to applicants to seek out this information and educate themselves on the steps. Applicants should also have done a great deal of reflecting about their motivation for medicine and been engaged in activities to support their motivation before moving forward with the application process.

Funding Medical School

To help applicants determine how to pay for medical school, the AAMC offers a great resource called Financial Information, Resources, Services, and Tools (FIRST) offering debt management, calculators, and toolkits. This can be found at https://students-residents.aamc.org/financial-aid/resources/.

Some medical schools offer scholarships while many applicants will fund their medical education via loans. Applicants who plan to use loans should submit a Free Application for Federal Student Aid (FAFSA) and have the information released to the medical school they will be attending. Medical schools will post their tuition rates on their websites.

Reflection from a Graduating Premedical Student

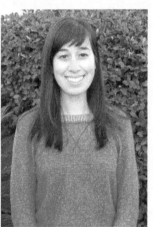

By Sara Fernandez
Vanderbilt University, BS, Child Development and
    Neuroscience, 2014
University of Texas Southwestern, Class of 2018

For me, I always considered completing the undergraduate pre-med curriculum as half of the battle in gaining admission to a medical school. After chemistry, biology, physics, and organic chemistry, the MCAT, the medical school applications, and the medical school interviews were still things that separated me from getting a seat in a medical school class.

In terms of studying for and taking the MCAT, that big first piece to your medical school application, all I can say is that you really have to give it your all. It takes time and perseverance to study for an exam that covers so much material, but do whatever you need to do to get in an environment where you can really focus. I know for me, MCAT studying required me to take over my parent's home office for a month and a half. MCAT preparation books, notes from my college courses, and scratch paper were spread everywhere, but this worked for me. This was my study zone, and when I needed a break, I could take one where I didn't have to look at anything relating to the MCAT. Little things like this helped me not to burn out.

After taking the MCAT, while waiting for my score report, I began to fill out my medical school applications. While applications for different schools may be formatted differently or have different essay prompts, there is definitely a consistency in terms of having to record any organizations, extracurriculars, or community service projects you were a part of throughout your entire undergraduate career. One thing I wish I would have done, and that I recommend you do, is make note of all the significant activities you do, as they happen, from the moment you begin your freshman year. All applications I completed asked for start dates and an estimation of the hours participated in each project, and doing this for an organization I was in during my first two years of college is somewhat tedious when you are a rising senior that has been away from that organization for a while. Recording things as they happen will save you time later! In terms of completing your application and reporting all those activities you were involved in, make sure you only put things down that you spent significant time on and that you are passionate about. For example, it is not worth reporting that you volunteered at a nursing home one summer if you only did so for an hour and a half of time. You will likely be asked about your activities, so make sure you have reported things you care about. If you are doing something just to fill your résumé, it will likely be apparent to the admissions committee and your interviewers.

I think one of the hardest things about the medical school application process is all the waiting involved. You must wait a month to get your MCAT score, you must wait for your application to be processed, you must wait to get interviews, and you must wait to hear about acceptances. All of this waiting is happening while you must go about your daily school or work routine, and sometimes it can be distracting. However, in terms of medical school applicants for a given year, you have to remember that you are just one of the thousands of students applying, and each student has many, many sheets of paper attached to them that must be looked at. In terms of the waiting, sometimes it caused me to second guess myself. *Had they chosen not to invite me to interview? Or had they just not gotten to my application yet?* I would often think about all the amazing students across the country I was competing with, and sometimes wish I had done things differently, but you have to remember that no one is perfect. There is no need to dwell on things that are done and think "Well, maybe if I would have made an A in that class rather than a B, I would have been invited for an interview already." You just have to remember that you tried your best, and what's done is done.

Once invitations to interview do come in, I think the process of visiting schools, meeting current students, and speaking with interviewers makes all the hard work put into applying worth it. It really does seem that most schools invite you to interview because they see something in you that they like, and this is something to be excited about! Before attending an interview, make sure you re-read your application and essays in case you are asked about them. Also, go ahead and look online at the school's website to see if there are any aspects of the school you may have questions about. Interviewers will always ask if you have questions for them, so it is good to be prepared with any you may have so you can leave your interview day feeling as if you know all you need to know about a medical school. Before my first interview, I thought I would only be interviewed by physicians, but throughout my interviews, I got to speak with great physicians, researchers, and admissions deans. This really allowed me to see how so many people associated with each medical school really care about your future development as a physician. At most schools you get to interact with current medical school students, and this is a great opportunity to ask about their experiences at that institution. Don't be shy. You could potentially be spending four years at this institution, and you want to know what your life could be like. Overall, I had assumed the interview process would be much more intimidating that it was. Really, it was exciting to picture myself being that much closer to becoming a physician!

Besides what I already mentioned above, demonstrating in your application and interview how you truly care about helping others will probably go the longest way! Best of luck!

Chapter 3 Worksheet

Activity Log

Build a log of activities since graduation from high school. This information will eventually be entered into the medical school application and will help you get a good start on keeping track of your activities.

Create a document (either Word or Excel) containing the following (since graduation from high school):

Academic Recognition (academic honors, awards, and other recognitions)

- Award Title
- Date Received
- City, State, Country
- Brief Description

Non-Academic Recognition

- Same as above

Leadership (leadership roles or positions of responsibility)

- Role Title
- Start/End Dates
- City, State, Country
- Brief Description

Employment (all paid jobs held since graduation from high school, including military service)

- Employer
- Job Title
- Start/End Dates
- City, State, Country
- Hours Worked per Week
- Brief Description of the Job

Research Activities (paid or volunteer)

- Research Activity Name
- Start/End Dates
- City, State, Country
- Approximate Hours per Week
- Brief Description

Health Care Activities (volunteer or paid)

- Activity Name
- Start/End Dates
- City, State, Country
- Hours per Week
- Total Cumulative Hours
- Brief Description

Community Service (non-health care related, volunteer only)

- Activity Name
- Start/End Dates
- City, State, Country
- Approximate Hours per Week
- Total Cumulative Hours
- Brief Description

Extracurricular & Leisure Activities

- Type of Activity
- Start/End Dates
- City, State, Country
- Approximate Hours per Month
- Total Cumulative Hours
- Brief Description

Chapter 3 Worksheet

Personal Statement

Using the worksheet from Chapter 2, which listed your reasons for wanting to pursue medicine, write a few paragraphs that begin to explain your motivation for pursuing a career as a physician. The application for medical school will require this essay.

Chapter 3 Worksheet

Health Care/Social Issues

When you interview for medical school, you will likely be asked about a current health care or social issue. In pursuing a career as a physician, it is important to begin to explore what issues are impacting the world.

Find one health care issue and one social issue that you find interesting. Answer the following:

Health Care Issue

- What is it?
- Why is it important in medicine?
- Why is it important to you?
- Are there any potential solutions?

Social Issue

- What is it?
- Why is it important in the world?
- Why is it important to you?
- Are there any potential solutions?

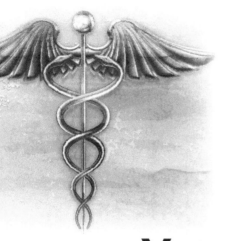

Chapter 4
Nontraditional/ Veteran/Military Applicants

Not everyone enrolling in medical school will begin straight out of college. Many applicants are applying after working in another field, serving in the military, or pursuing a graduate degree. Although Chapter 3 covers many aspects that will also apply to these applicants, this chapter will cover topics specifically for nontraditional applicants.

What Makes an Applicant Nontraditional?

There are many ways applicants are defined as nontraditional. Typically, a traditional applicant is one who pursued college straight out of high school and applies to medical school during their final year of college. If the applicant successfully gains admission on the first application, they matriculate into medical school a few months after completing their baccalaureate degrees. Nontraditional applicants, however, often pursue very different pathways. Below are some of the more common examples of nontraditional applicants.

- *Career or employment history*—This includes people who were employed for a period of time *outside* of the time they were enrolled in undergraduate studies.
  - This might include individuals who worked following high school. After more than a year (sometimes several), they may have decided to pursue a baccalaureate degree. They may then gain admission immediately after earning their degree, but since they were in the workforce prior to college, they may be considered nontraditional due to age and experience outside of higher education.

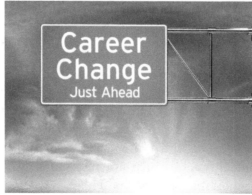

© Digital Storm/Shutterstock.com

○ The other group is those who earn their undergraduate degree in a different field, pursuing work in that field (or unrelated employment) for a time. Once they decide they want to pursue medicine, this group may then take medical school prerequisites (either full-time or part-time while continuing to work).

- *Graduate degrees*—Sometimes people decide to pursue graduate degrees (either master or doctoral level) before they decide to pursue medicine. This decision may be made to prepare them for medicine or it may have been unrelated.

- *Military history*—Those who have served as active duty military personnel will have served a minimum number of years. These individuals may have earned a baccalaureate degree during their service or when they discharged from the military, while others may be in the officer ranks. This group will be covered in more detail below.

- *Age*—Applicants who are 25 years old or older at the time of matriculation are often considered nontraditional. Clearly, these individuals will fall into one or several of the above categories. Age is not a factor that is used in determining admission. It is simply used here to explain, in years, who may be considered in this category.

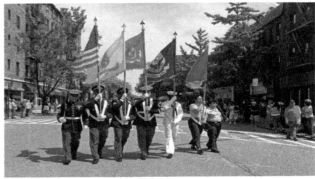

© a katz/Shutterstock.com

Advising

Nontraditional individuals often have not had any direct advising for preparing for medical school since their pathway may not have easily put them in touch with the premedical advising process. The only groups that may be able to utilize premedical advising are those who pursue a baccalaureate degree after some time spent in employment. Since these people are pursuing their degree at an institution that will likely have a premedical advisor or office, they can take advantage of the same assistance as a traditional student. People who fall into every other category may find themselves navigating the preparation-phase and application-process solo. This need not be the case. It will be important for individuals like this to seek advice from medical school admissions officers and application services and utilize resources like this book. There are many nuances to the preparation-phase, so it will be important for these individuals to determine a timeline for completing the necessary steps.

Postbaccalaureate Programs and Graduate Degrees

In some cases it will be important for an applicant to consider taking courses following their undergraduate years. This is often the case for applicants who have a less than average academic record, earned lower grades in their science coursework, or did not pursue science coursework in undergraduate school.

One way of remedying a poor academic record, especially a science record, is to attend a postbaccalaureate program or earn a graduate degree in a basic science area. Some of these programs are designed to help the applicant be more academically competitive for medical school and also serve the purpose of providing a solid foundation for the entrance into medical school.

The AAMC offers a searchable database for postbaccalaureate programs throughout the nation: *https://apps.aamc.org/postbac/#/index*. In the state of Texas, there is a one-year Master of Science in Medical Science program offered through the Graduate School of Biomedical Sciences at the University of North Texas Health Science Center: *https://www.unthsc.edu/graduate-school-of-biomedical-sciences/formerly-the-post-baccalaureate-premedical-program/*.

There is also a postbaccalaureate certification program at the University of Texas at Dallas: *http://www.utdallas.edu/pre-health/post-bacc-studies*. This program is geared toward someone who already has a bachelor's degree but needs to take the prerequisite courses.

It may be helpful to first seek advising from a prehealth advisor or a medical school advisor as to whether pursuing a postbaccalaureate or master's degree is the best option for the situation.

Coursework

Depending on each individual situation, applicants who find that it has been several years since they took any coursework (including the prerequisite courses) or were a full-time student may benefit from pursuing one of the options mentioned above. It will be important for the applicant to verify with each medical school they intend to apply to whether the prerequisite courses "expire" or must be taken within a certain timeframe before applying. Some medical schools have no expiration date for coursework, however, admissions committees may want to see that the prerequisite courses were taken recently and/or that an applicant was a full-time student in the recent past to be better prepared for the preclinical years of medical school.

Academic Fresh Start

In the state of Texas, there is a program called Academic Fresh Start that keeps older college grades from counting against the grade point average (GPA). This may be an option for an applicant who has coursework that is 10 or more years old with a lower GPA that may hinder the chances of gaining admission to medical school. Through Academic Fresh Start, coursework that is 10 years old and older is cleared from the academic record. This means that those grades are not calculated into the GPA, nor are the credits used toward a degree. Some key points to keep in mind:

- You cannot choose which courses are kept. ALL coursework that is 10 years old and older is cleared from the academic record.
- You may have to retake prerequisite coursework even if you had previously performed well.
- You may have to retake courses to complete a new degree if they were party of the group that was cleared. You do not lose any previously earned degrees.
- It may help your GPA tremendously when you apply to medical school as the GPA earned prior to Academic Fresh Start will not be used in the evaluation process. There is a question on the TMDSAS application that asks about Academic Fresh Start.

This may be a great option for some applicants. Also keep in mind that in Texas, the requirement to qualify for entry into medical school is 90 semester credit hours. If an applicant has enrolled through Academic Fresh Start and takes 90 semester credit hours or has some coursework that was newer than 10 years to count, he/she may not have to actually earn another degree. It will be very important to speak to a prehealth advisor or medical school admissions Dean or Director for feedback to determine if this is the right path. For more information about Academic Fresh Start, visit http://www.collegeforalltexans.com/index.cfm?objectid=6D10C9BD-DD24-153F-90B91DA6C20D1C97.

Letters of Recommendation/Evaluation

This section was covered in the previous chapter but it is important to touch on a few unique points for nontraditional applicants. As stated previously in this chapter, applicants may not have access to a premedical advising office/advisor as they will often be out of the traditional pipeline. If this is the case, it is important to check with each admissions office (may also be detailed on the application services' websites) to verify whom letters should come from. Most traditional applicants will have letters from their current or most recent professors, research mentors, college/university organization advisors, or health professions advisory committees. Nontraditional applicants may be better served by requesting their letters from employment supervisors, military commanding officers or superiors, physicians shadowed, or other professional contacts. When possible, it would be beneficial to a nontraditional applicant to obtain one letter from a science faculty member (if the coursework was completed recently).

Military/Veteran Applicants

Those who are on active duty in the military at the time of application or have completed their military commitments have unique circumstances for consideration in the application process. Their pathways may include coursework taken from multiple institutions over an extended period of time, experiences

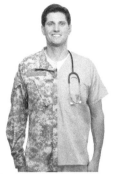 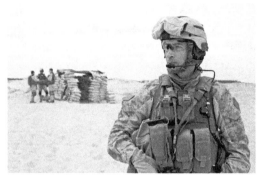

© Straight 8 Photography/Shutterstock.com   © Oleg Zabielin/Shutterstock.com

with deployment, leadership opportunities, and adjustments to living in multiple locations and environments. These unique experiences help military/veteran applicants stand out.

Each application will provide an opportunity to list military history and current status. If possible, it may also be beneficial to discuss some of the unique opportunities and experiences obtained while in service in an essay and/or under leadership.

Coursework

Since active duty military personnel are working full-time, sometimes on deployment or other mission-related duties, they may be taking courses to earn their baccalaureate degree or to fulfill the prerequisite curriculum for entry into medical school while at different locations. This may mean that the coursework was taken at different institutions or online. It is important to ensure that the courses are taken from regionally accredited institutions. It may also be helpful to include in the application an explanation as to why this was necessary. These applicants should not make the assumption that medical school faculty/admissions officers will have knowledge or experience with military circumstances, so it is best to explain why this is the case.

Leadership and Other Unique Experiences

Applicants should highlight and include the unique experiences gained from serving in the military. These applicants will often have unique leadership or training experiences that set them apart from other applicants. When the applications allow for these experiences to be entered, applicants should include them. When that is not possible, they can find a way to talk about them in their essay(s).

Advising

Since there will likely not be an opportunity to seek formal premedical advising for these applicants, they should seek the assistance from medical school admissions officers at schools where they will be applying. If they come across resistance or discouragement, they should continue until they find someone who will work to understand their specific circumstances. There are admissions officers who are happy to help these unique applicants and see them as an enriching addition to the medical school class. This advising is also helpful in determining the best way to approach the application, which experiences to share, and how to round out their experiences if there are any weaknesses.

Diversity

Whether nontraditional applicants realize it or not, they will enhance the learning of their medical school classmates. They bring unique characteristics and experiences to the classroom that many of their traditional classmates may not have had. These individuals bring diversity to medicine as well which may help them relate differently with patients. Applicants should not view their status of "nontraditional" as a detriment to the process, but instead as an added value.

Reflection from a Former Accountant

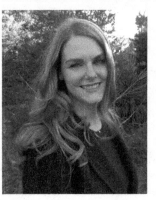

By Danielle Black
University of the Incarnate Word, BBA, 2007,
    Summa Cum Laude
University of the Incarnate Word, MSA, 2009,
    Summa Cum Laude
University of Texas at San Antonio,
    Post-Baccalaureate Studies,
    2011–2013
Texas A&M Health Science Center College of
    Medicine, Class of 2018

Self-doubt has always been the monster under my bed. It took a year to brave a career change, and sending the TMDSAS and AMCAS primary applications was so gut wrenching that I proofread them for two weeks before clicking submit. If uncertainty is among your struggles as you apply to medical school, you are not alone. In my opinion, the most important indicator of success in any profession is the earnest desire to pursue that path. Build that framework first, and the rest falls into place as each action and experience bolsters your future endeavors.

Other non-traditional pre-medical students I have met along the way confirm that many grapple with "fear of failure" or a reluctance to take the leap. Medicine's barriers to entry are formidable, with special emphasis placed on statistics and performance on high-stakes exams in a way that often seems biased and unfair. Every serious pre-medical student agonizes over essays, character allowances, which experiences to highlight, and interview preparation. The application process, from the MCAT through interview season, humbles you until your response to, "Where do you want to do go to medical school?" is a squeaky, "Anywhere that will take me! You won't believe the amazing people I met on my last interview."

There was a time when I embraced the possibility of not gaining acceptance. Strangely, even with the prospect of having to apply again next cycle, I was still much happier than as a disgruntled accountant trying to ignore the fact that I was in the wrong profession. For many years, when I spoke of my studies or career I was forced to endure, without inspiration, the tired, "So you're a bean counter, huh?" My choice to study accounting at twenty years of age was driven entirely by practicality under a misguided plan to secure a life for myself first and soul search at a later time. I pushed forward with the sincere thought that working hard on something, anything, would result in a revelation of the "perfect" life and career later—always later. With no clear idea of my definition of perfection, this blind scramble was even more unsound.

By the time I had a graduate degree and a CPA license, I thought I had travelled too far down the road to turn back. One day I realized a third of my life was over and changed my attitude about finding my life's work. A career switch is not turning back, it is simply taking a different trail up the mountain. I quit my accounting job and packed a backpack to work in outdoor recreation for two years as an adventure trip leader, climbing instructor, team building facilitator, and counselor for at-risk youth throughout the United States. The literal mountains I climbed were emotional parallels of the mountains I was climbing inside.

I envy those who have known their purpose in life from a young age, but do not despair if you are not one of those few. My best advice to all pre-medical students, or anyone at all, is to mine your life's gem and polish it. Wherever your interests lie, the only real failure is to give up searching for what will unleash your unique combination of abilities on the world, even if that means failure or embarrassment. It is not the world's responsibility to show us what our highest and best use to society will be; it is our own job to hear our inner voice and then strive to reach our potential. Life is an ungraded exam, but I want to be able to say at the end that I gave it my absolute all.

The instant I committed to entering the field of medicine I woke up each morning like a warrior. The attempt became the adventure, and the path was validated when the journey itself became exciting. My results exceeded expectations when I stopped focusing on the end-game and became present; even the most basic science courses filled my cup. Suddenly schoolwork, volunteering, shadowing, and three jobs became a feasible challenge, although my schedule appeared nearly impossible to others. Naysayers' snarky comments rolled off my back as they never had before. I fell into bed each night happier than I had been in years! I even found a social niche I did not know existed as I met others pursuing the same dream. Finding the right career must be like falling in love; you know when it is right.

My first interview was terrifying, but I quickly realized that admissions committees and interviewers are just normal folks who have the important task of promoting their institution. They may spill their drinks, take phone calls in the middle of your interview, or ask marginally inappropriate questions. Extend to them the same grace you would expect, but keep in mind that they are just as fallible as you are. Interviews quickly became my favorite part of the application process. Use them to meet your future mentors and colleagues, marvel at the accomplishments of your fellow applicants, and let your heart, smile, and love shine. The applicants who are so excited about medical school that they could burst are obvious. I assure you that if every day since you decided to become a doctor reflects your strength of conviction for medicine as a calling, Admissions will see you.

Soon I will join the Class of 2018 at Texas A&M Health Science Center in Temple, TX, to begin a decade of training and a lifetime of learning. I am ecstatic to spend every day side by side with some of the most talented and charismatic people I have ever met. The chance to someday be a healer, resource, and teacher for those searching for health and well-being makes the entire process more than worth it! I promise.

Reflection from an Army Veteran

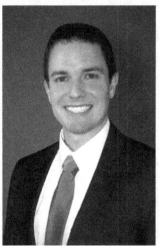

By Matthew Vassaur
Texas A&M University, Bachelor of Arts: Spanish,
Class of 2008
Texas A&M Health Science Center
College of Medicine, Class of 2018
Former Army Captain, 4.5 Years of Active Duty
Served

Deciding to pursue medicine is intimidating for anyone, but it is particularly daunting for nontraditional or military applicants. The logistics of relocating a family, the necessary financial sacrifices, and the relational strains caused by the demands of medicine are all reasons that many nontraditional applicants forgo a career in medicine. These are legitimate concerns, and I fault no one who determines that the sacrifices are too great to pursue this journey, but for those who are truly called to medicine I wish to offer my perspective.

I served as an officer in the US Army from 2008 to 2012 after graduating from Texas A&M University with a degree in Spanish language. I entered school as a premedical student, but after 1 year of struggling to balance the demands of the Corps of Cadets and my basic science courses, I changed majors to focus on preparing to enter military service. My experiences in the Army were like many others who entered at a similar time; our nation was at war, and I had the distinct honor of leading Soldiers overseas. Those 12 months I spent serving in the Middle East were crucial to my decision to become a physician, though I was not aware of it at the time. Most of my responsibilities were looking after those under my command and making decisions with potentially life and death consequences. Safeguarding the well-being of others offered me a degree of fulfillment that I had never experienced before, which laid the foundation that would eventually lead me back to medicine.

After earning the rank of Captain many exciting career opportunities opened up for me, and I was anxious to tackle greater challenges in the military. One opportunity that played a pivotal role in leading me to medicine was being afforded the chance to attend the US Army Pathfinder School. Pathfinders are elite troops with a lineage dating back to World War II where they prepared drop zones for US forces jumping into Europe and the Pacific. All those who attend the school are individually selected and of those roughly half fail to complete the course. Successful completion of the training requires tremendous discipline and around the clock studying for 3 weeks to pass the constant barrage of examinations. I put forth my best effort and, fortunately, I was rewarded with the coveted Pathfinder torch. Though more importantly, I achieved a great sense of satisfaction at facing a formidable challenge and I learned that I actually *enjoyed* studying for so many long hours. While unaware of it at the time, that truth would prove to be an important component of the decision that I would make several months later.

In the relaxing setting of a warm beach on a family vacation I was speaking with my brother, a first year medical student at the Texas A&M Health Science Center (TAMHSC), and inquired about the demands of medical school. I asked him to outline his day and detail the hours he spent studying, which I realized were remarkably similar to my own schedule in Pathfinder School. Although my material was not as intricate, a flicker of hope flashed inside of me and I began to wonder if I, too, had the makings of a future physician. However, that hope died quickly when I remembered my own struggles in freshman-level Chemistry. After continued discussion about medical school my brother could sense not only my intrigue, but also my own self-doubt.

He looked me in the eye and said, "Matt, we're brothers. If I can do it, you can do it too." Having someone of his experience express certainty in my intelligence was all the convincing I needed. Within 1 hour of talking to him about the details of premedical studies I was anxious to drop the status that I had built in the military and pursue what I felt God to be calling me toward, a career in medicine.

Once my mind was made up, everything after that happened in rapid succession. Within 5 months of learning what the Lord had in store for me professionally, I was out of the military and taking my first premedical class in nearly 8 years. However, getting there was not easy, and it involved a lot of legwork. My very first move was to make an exhaustive list of pros and cons for following medicine or staying in the military. Sure, I had my moment on the beach where I felt the Lord calling me to medicine, but in order to know for sure, I scrutinized every detail of my plan, mapped out the next 10 years of my life (including the ramifications for my family), and discussed it all at length with my wife. Once we had determined that pursuing medicine was the best move for our family and for my own personal fulfillment, the next step was to get a professional mentor.

Realizing that gaining admittance into an American medical school is one of the hardest scholastic goals one can achieve is an important truth to accept. Consequently, it is vital to speak with someone who specializes in counseling premedical students. The two professionals I sought out were my undergraduate premedical advisor and Leila Diaz, a key member of the admissions committee at the TAMHSC and one of the authors of this book. As I learned, Leila not only was a highly respected member of the admissions committee, but was also an advocate for military veterans. Having worked extensively with many veterans pursuing medicine, Leila was better able to understand my background than most. The jargon alone of military service can be extremely difficult to translate to civilian terms, so anyone already familiar with military applicants can be tremendously helpful. Leila has proven instrumental to my own success and I advise any veteran pursuing medicine to contact a medical school admissions committee and inquire about a specific point of contact for military veteran applicants.

Having established contact with two professional advisors I was directed to a state university that offered a "postbaccalaureate" program for nontraditional students seeking to become healthcare professionals. Though the application deadline had already passed, I emailed the head of the program who waived the deadline, and I was granted acceptance. From there, I went head on in my studies by signing up for a full load of science courses and treated school as a full-time job. By applying the discipline that I learned in the military and dedicating the level of attention required for premedical courses, I was able to excel and 2 years later I am a first-year medical student at my alma mater, Texas A&M University!

My perspective is that of a veteran who discovered medicine in his late twenties, but the core of my story applies to anyone and goes beyond the pursuit of medicine. In truth, one's intelligence is only half of the equation, and being afforded the privilege to study medicine is more a function of self-belief, discipline, and desire. Self-belief leads to the removal of the invisible chains and limitations that we place on ourselves, and allows us to envision a dream that is worth pursuing. The fundamental difference between me as an 18-year-old freshman struggling in his introductory science courses and the first-year medical student that I am today is the fact that I dared to believe my brother's confidence in my abilities and have dedicated myself to proving him right. I am still on the journey to achieving my dream, but I am certain that I will succeed. So to anyone reading this, I implore you to place full confidence in your ability to attain your own dream and dare to have the courage to pursue it, you will be amazed by what is possible.

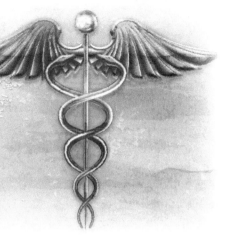

Chapter 5
Osteopathic Medicine and Allopathic Medicine

Many aspiring doctors do not initially recognize that there are two distinct degrees that grant the right to practice as a physician: Medical Doctor (MD) and Doctor of Osteopathic Medicine (DO). The MD degree has been available longer and there are more MD medical schools than DO schools, however the DO profession is rapidly growing with

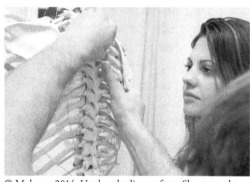

© Mahony, 2014. Used under license from Shutterstock, Inc.

more and more medical schools available nationwide. Both are fully licensed physicians, trained in diagnosing and treating illness and providing health care. Both prescribe medication, perform surgery, and practice in all specialty areas.

Allopathic Medicine

Allopathy is a term coined by C. F. S. Hahnemann (founder of homeopathy) in 1842 to describe mainstream medicine and defined it as "the system of medical practice which treats disease by the use of remedies which produce effects different from those produced by the diseases under treatment" (www .medterms.com). This term is not widely used today by MDs except in comparison with osteopathic medicine and its use is discouraged by others (Katherine E. Gundling, MD, "When Did I Become an 'Allopath'?" *Archives of Internal Medicine* 158, no. 20 [November 1998]: 2185–2186).

Generally, physicians are distinguished as either having an MD (allopathic medicine) or DO (osteopathic medicine). The training is almost identical with the exception of an additional treatment modality DOs are trained in and a philosophy of medicine (described below).

The term "osteopathy" alone is discouraged when referring to DOs. The AOA (American Osteopathic Association) encourages the use of "osteopathic medicine" to refer to fully licensed physicians who graduated from osteopathic medical schools in the United States (http://www.osteopathic.org/inside-aoa/ news-and-publications/media-center/Pages/osteopathic-style-guide.aspx).

Osteopathic Medicine

In 1874, an MD physician, Andrew T. Still, founded osteopathic medicine. The philosophy of holistic medicine focused on treating illness within the context of the whole body (www.aacom.org/become-a-doctor/about-om/history). He taught that the systems of the body were interrelated and impacted one another supporting the idea to treat illness within a broader context and to focus on preventative care. Interestingly, the principles of holistic medicine and preventative care are also taught within MD schools. Osteopathic medicine has grown since it was founded, amounting to 34 accredited DO schools as of 2017 (www.aacom.org). There are more than 74,000 DOs practicing in the United States (www.aacom.org/become-a-doctor/about-om/history). Interestingly, the principles of holistic medicine and preventative care are also taught within MD schools.

DOs are trained in all of the same aspects of medicine as MDs and can be licensed to practice in all fifty states. Graduates of osteopathic medical programs may pursue residencies in either osteopathic or allopathic programs in all specialties of medicine. While in medical school, DOs additionally learn a treatment modality called Osteopathic Manipulative Medicine (OMM). OMM is a set of manual manipulation techniques involving the musculoskeletal system, which DOs can use to diagnose illness, restore range of motion, and enhance the body's natural tendency toward self-healing (www.aacom.org/become-a-doctor/about-om/history).

Curricular Similarities and Differences

Traditionally, there is only one main curricular difference between allopathic and osteopathic medical schools. Osteopathic medical students will often take an additional course throughout medical school in OMM. This is the main modality that makes DOs different from their MD counterparts. DO students will learn the science behind OMM and how to perform the various functions of the treatment modality. In addition to the course, DO students will also have an OMM rotation in their clinical years utilizing this treatment with patients. Some DOs will go on to specialize in OMM. There is also an opportunity for either DO or MD graduates to participate in an OMM Fellowship.

Board Examinations

As described later in *Chapter 8: Medical School Curriculum Clinical Years*, both MD and DO students will take board exams during their 2nd and 4th years of medical school. These exams are similar, however they are scored differently. Because of the scoring difference and because DO students may want to apply to MD residencies, many DO students will take the USMLE in addition to their COMLEX exams. This allows them to report both scores when applying to residency and demonstrate that their application is competitive to residency programs that are not accustomed to reviewing COMLEX scores.

USMLE Steps and COMLEX Levels

MD students will take a 3-part board exam called the United States Medical Licensing Examination (USMLE). DO students will also take a 3-part board exam called the Comprehensive Osteopathic Medical Licensing Examination (COMLEX).

The USMLE has three steps taken at different points within the medical training. Successful completion of these exams allows a physician to practice medicine without supervision. It is composed of the following (http://www .usmle.org):

- USMLE Step 1 (taken at the end of the 2nd year of medical school): Assess a student's knowledge and ability to apply important concepts in basic sciences, with an emphasis on principles and mechanisms of disease and modes of therapy.
- USMLE Step 2 Clinical Knowledge (taken at the beginning of the 4th year of medical school): Assesses the student's ability to apply medical knowledge, skills, and understanding of clinical science to providing patient care.
- USMLE Step 2 Clinical Skills: Assesses the student's mastery of clinical skills tested in a standardized patient[*] setting.
- USMLE Step 3 (taken during residency): Assesses the ability to apply medical knowledge and understanding of biomedical and clinical sciences to unsupervised practice of medicine with an emphasis on patient management in ambulatory settings.

The COMLEX sequence is comparable to the USMLE in regards to when the steps are taken. It is composed of the following (https://www.nbome .org/candidates.asp?m=can):

- COMLEX Level 1: Assesses basic science knowledge as it applies to medical problems emphasizing the scientific concepts and principles necessary for understanding mechanisms of health, medical problems, and disease processes.
- COMLEX Level 2 Cognitive Evaluation: Demonstrate knowledge of clinical concepts and medical decision-making.
- COMLEX Level 2 Performance Evaluation: Assesses knowledge in three areas—Patient Presentation, Osteopathic Medical Practice, and Clinical Content.
- COMLEX Level 3: Demonstrate knowledge of clinical concepts and principles necessary for solving medical problems independently.

Residency Programs

Previously, DO students applied to DO residencies and matched to a residency through the American Osteopathic Association (AOA) or to an MD residency

---

[*]Standardized patients are trained actors who act out symptoms and use a scripted dialogue.

through the National Resident Matching Program (NRMP). MD students only applied to residencies through the NRMP.

In 2014, the Accreditation Council for Graduate Medical Education (ACGME), the American Osteopathic Association (AOA), and the American Association of Colleges of Osteopathic Medicine (AACOM) agreed to a single accreditation system for graduate medical education (GME) or what is known as residency training. This means that graduates of both allopathic and osteopathic medical schools will complete their residency and/or fellowship education in ACGME-accredited programs and achieve common milestones and competencies http://www.osteopathic.org/inside-aoa/single-gme-accreditation -system/Pages/default.aspx. Once AOA-approved programs receive ACGME accreditation (anticipated completion of 2020), it will open more opportunities for all graduating medical students to apply to more programs as well as incoporate osteopathic principles into the ACGME framework (https://www.aamc .org/newsroom/reporter/june2014/384802/gme.html). Both are eligible to join and match to a residency through the military.

Choosing

Applicants deciding whether to apply to MD and/or DO medical schools should shadow and talk with physicians in both fields. Just as in the general plan to choose which medical schools to apply to, applicants should research the particulars of what each medical school's focus is, how the curriculum is taught, the average MCAT and GPA for admitted students, and other admissions requirements, success of students on board exams and residency placement, and overall culture of the school. All of this data, regardless if it is an MD or DO school, will help inform the applicant's choice.

Reflection from a DO Physician

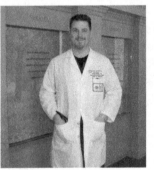

By Heath D. White, DO, MS
Director, Medical Intensive Care Unit, 2016-present
Attending Physician, Division of Pulmonary,
*   Critical Care & Sleep Medicine, Baylor Scott*
*   & White Healthcare, 2012–present*
Assistant Professor, Texas A&M Health Science
*   Center, College of Medicine, 2012–present*
Lung Transplantation and Interventional Pulmonology
*   Fellowship, University of Texas at San Antonio,*
*   San Antonio, TX, 2011–2012*
Pulmonary and Critical Care Medicine Fellowship,
*   Scott & White Memorial Hospital, Temple, TX,*
*   2008–2011*
Internal Medicine Residency, Scott & White Memorial Hospital, Temple, TX,
*   2005–2008*
Doctor of Osteopathic Medicine, University of North Texas Health Science Center,
*   Texas College of Osteopathic Medicine, 2005*
Master of Science, University of North Texas Health Science Center, 2005
*   Bachelor of Science, Baylor University, 2000*

When applying to medical school, the goal is the same no matter where you choose to apply. That goal is to become a physician and that's the simple truth. Now, there are two routes to become a physician: allopathic medicine and osteopathic medicine, MD and DO. So how do you choose? Do you need to choose? What's the difference? These are questions that have to be answered as you begin your application process.

When I look at my medical career in reflection, these were questions that I asked myself during the application process. At that time, the questions did not personally matter to me and the answer to those questions was always simply a statement of my career goal—I want to be a physician. Now when I reflect on these questions, I actually have answers and the answers have meaning to me as a person and as a physician. The answers to those questions have helped define me as a physician, given me confidence in my profession, and have provided me with goals far beyond my initial ambitions of "becoming a physician."

Osteopathic medicine was founded in the late 1800s and is now well recognized within the field of medicine. The difference between MDs and DOs has been blurred over time for a variety of reasons, but the philosophic principles of osteopathic medicine as A. T. Still originally described them remain the backbone behind osteopathic principles and practice to date. The osteopathic approach to medicine includes all those things that would be defined as traditional medicine (prescriptions, surgeries, and evidence-based medicine), but what many do not take into account and appreciate is the additional things that Osteopathic Medicine offers. A core osteopathic principle is that the body is a unit with the innate ability to heal itself and provide self-regulation. With this comes a direct relationship between body structure and function, which is where Osteopathic Manipulative Medicine plays a role.

What does all this mean for an aspiring medical student with that one goal in mind? To most of the aspiring students, I suspect it doesn't mean much. To me, I think it means a lot. This was important when I was a medical student because I had to learn this to become a physician. Now . . . it guides me in my treatment of each and every patient by providing the big picture view and addressing the "elephant in the room." How does one system relate to the other and how can I address each of these problems to fix the big picture?

My goals upon entering medical school were pretty clear-cut to me when I started. Finish medical school, do a residency in family medicine, and go back to my hometown and be the local physician. I planned on being that small town primary care physician. So what did I do instead . . . extend medical school to five years and combine it with a Master of Science in Clinical Research and Education and a pre-doctoral fellowship in Osteopathic Manipulative Medicine (OMM), complete a residency in Internal Medicine, followed by a fellowship in Pulmonary & Critical Care Medicine, and then complete a fellowship in Lung Transplantation and Interventional Pulmonology. And to complete the reversal of my original plans, I now practice in an academic tertiary care referral center. All of my post-graduate training was completed in allopathic programs.

Many students will change their goals throughout medical school and post-graduate training. In regards to my original plan, osteopathic medicine is well-known for its training of primary care physicians and their numbers support that hands down, but it also provides the opportunity to train in any specialty of medicine. My plans changed multiple times during the course of medical school just as numerous students and trainees do.

Each step that I have made since starting medical school has taught me something unique and I attribute that to the philosophic backbone of osteopathic principles. I believe in the osteopathic principles and holistic approach but I also believe in evidence-based medicine. The combined education of osteopathic principles, OMM,

continued

Reflection from a DO Physician *(continued)*

and "traditional medicine" has not only influenced my day-to-day approach to treatment but it has also opened numerous doors along the way through my education. The choices I have made with graduate work and multiple post-graduate training opportunities have all been influenced by my osteopathic medical education and my current practice would not be the same without that education.

Decisions are always easier to make in retrospect. Sometimes you make the right one and sometimes the wrong one. I chose to be a DO because that is the school where I was accepted. My knowledge of osteopathic medicine in the application process was really no more than the ability to rehash the osteopathic principles for the purpose of an interview. But if I were to do this over again with the choice, would I choose the same path . . . hands down without a reservation.

I end with a quote: "Life moves pretty fast. If you don't stop and look around once in a while, you could miss it."—Ferris Bueller, *Ferris Bueller's Day Off*

Stop, look, and research your choices. My choice has furthered me as a professional and a person. Let your decisions not be made in retrospect.

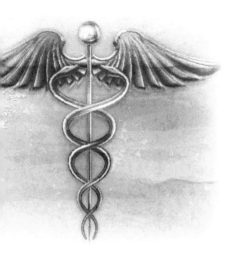

Chapter 6
Joint Degree Medical Programs

Students will have the opportunity to pursue more than their MD or DO degrees while in medical school. Many medical schools offer the opportunity to pursue other fields of study in conjunction with the medical degree. Just like deciding to pursue medicine, students need to explore and gain some exposure in these fields to ensure it is an

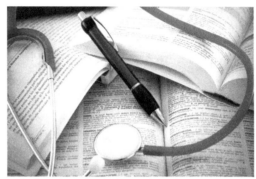

© dauf, 2014. Used under license from Shutterstock, Inc.

additional educational pursuit they want to engage in and they have a realistic understanding of how it may be applied to and fit in with their career as a physician. Most of the programs will have their own application process, entrance exam requirements, and extracurricular activities such as research or internships that they emphasize.

Master's Degrees

The option for a master's degree will often only add 1–2 extra years to the student's overall undergraduate medical education training. Below are the most commonly pursued as a dual option.

Master of Public Health

Many medical schools operate within a health science center that has other health professions colleges often including a school of public health. A Master of Public Health (MPH) is a degree that fits nicely with the study of medicine. This degree usually adds only one additional year to the standard four years of medical school. The MPH will

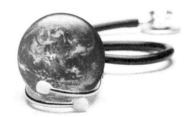

© Fordon Saunders, 2014. Used under license from Shutterstock, Inc.

likely provide various concentrations for the student to choose such as health policy, epidemiology, global health, and environmental health. Public health focuses on the broader context of health including the community at-large whereas medicine often focuses on the individual patient. Obtaining an MPH degree may prepare the future physician for work in specific communities, within state or local government contributing to health policy, global health, conducting research, focusing on population health, or implementing community-wide (or larger) programs.

Master of Science

If the student is interested in research, has contributed to research during his/her undergraduate years, and would like to incorporate it into the career as a physician, the Master of Science (MS) may be an option. In addition to science course work in the subfield the student has selected, an MS will also include research. The research is presented at the end of the degree in a thesis, which the student must present before their committee. Typically, a student would pursue an MS rather than a PhD if they envision their career incorporating some research pursuits but their clinical practice still being the focus.

Master of Science in Clinical and Translational Science is another science-based masters offered at several medical schools. This dual degree serves to train future physicians to combine their clinical knowledge with the skills needed to conduct and direct research preparing them for a career as clinical researchers.

Master of Business Administration

The Master of Business Administration (MBA) may seem unfitting with a career in medicine; however, students who have taken business classes in college may see how an MBA could be applied to a career in medicine. A student who is interested in health government work, health policy, hospital or health care administration, and/or industry work (biotechnology, pharmaceuticals, and medical devices) in their career would greatly benefit from an MBA. Also, many physicians will choose to practice in a private clinic, either alone or with other physician partners, therefore, the backing of a business degree would certainly be useful.

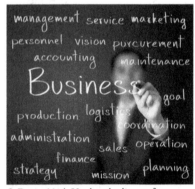

© Dusit, 2014. Used under license from Shutterstock, Inc.

Master of Science Education for Health Care Professionals

Some medical schools offer the opportunity for dual degree master-level programs focused on preparing students to work as teachers, leaders, and/or administrators at the medical school or residency training level. These degrees will help train students to be teachers in their specific field of medicine, conduct research, serve as administrators involved in leadership and/or curriculum development, and/or develop innovative educational programs in medical education.

Other Masters

Various medical schools offer other options for master-level dual degrees. Some may include a Master in Divinity (MDiv), Master of Health Science (MHS), Master of Public Administration (MPA), Master of Social Work (MSW), and others.

Doctoral Degrees

There are a handful of medical school applicants who know they want a more advanced dual focus in their career and choose to pursue a second doctoral degree along with their medical degree. The two most common doctoral dual degree programs are research and law.

Doctor of Philosophy

Students who have been heavily engaged in research during their college years and wish to include research in their career as a physician, balancing patient care and research, or focusing primarily on research, might consider a PhD and become a "physician-scientist." The MD/PhD or DO/PhD is probably the most common dual degree offered at medical schools. The PhD dual degree will likely add three to six years in addition to the four years of medical school.

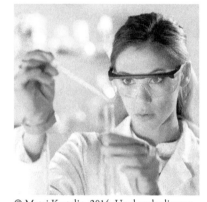

© Matej Kastelic, 2014. Used under license from Shutterstock, Inc.

Due to the large commitment needed to complete this dual degree, students should engage in lengthy research projects during undergraduate school where they have an active role in conducting research. This exposure is necessary to not only decide if this would be the right career path, but also determine the kind of research one would be interested in pursuing during the PhD portion of their training, and the kind of research they envision conducting in their career. A well thought-out plan backed by experience will be necessary to be competitive for one of these positions.

Doctor of Jurisprudence

Students who envision a career within health law and/or policy, forensics, or biomedical compliance may consider a law degree in conjunction with their MD or DO. A JD degree may also benefit someone who is interested in teaching medical students and/or residents about health law or serving as a medical school or hospital administrator. Similar to other dual degrees, students need to thoroughly explore whether this would be a good option. Students should gain some exposure to law careers and research the educational pathway. Students need to have a well-defined idea and perspective of why they chose to pursue an MD/JD dual degree. JD degrees in conjunction with the MD typically add another two years to the standard four years of medical school for six years total (one year less than the degrees acquired separately).

Benefit/Value of a Dual Degree

Dual degrees allow a future physician to add an additional component to their career. In addition to seeing patients, physicians may want to be heavily involved in research, work within educational, hospital, or governmental administration, or focus on the broader community and education.

Having additional training may also help the student be more competitive for residencies that are more difficult to get into. Some residencies value exposure that comes from some of these dual degrees. However, students should be careful not to pursue an additional degree they are not interested in just to be more competitive for residency. Added training may also open up career opportunities in their future.

Similar to medicine, students should only pursue these degrees if they have researched them and gained some preliminary experience in the area they are interested in. This will help them make an informed decision about whether they are fitting for their career goals. This will require them to have a better idea of what they envision their career in medicine to entail. Dual degrees will add additional time and debt to the training period so it should not be a decision made lightly. Physicians can also pursue these additional degrees after their medical careers have been established.

Reflection from an MD, PhD

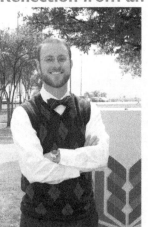

By John Reneau, MD, PhD
Texas A&M Health Science Center College of Medicine,
  Class of 2013
Residency: Internal Medicine, Mayo School of Graduate
  Medical Education, Rochester, MN

When I began the application process for medical school, I had already done a significant amount of clinical research during college. Having enjoyed the research environment, I pursued a combined MD/PhD program thinking it would be a great fit for me. The experience has been very challenging, yet rewarding. Two of the more difficult aspects of combined degree training are the length of time it takes to complete and the vast differences between clinical and research training.

The extra years of training for a doctoral degree may not seem like a lot when you are applying, but once you begin on the path you may feel differently. Breaking away from your friends and colleagues to pursue research as they finish medical school and graduate can be emotionally draining and very demoralizing. I remember going to the graduation for the medical school class with which I entered and thinking, "Wow . . . I could be graduating right now, but instead I'm stuck in a lab running the same experiments over and over and I still can't get them to work." I did eventually get the experiments working, but that moment helped put into perspective that PhD training does take a significant amount of time and this is worthwhile considering as you are applying. It is reasonable to expect to spend no less than three years pursuing research, but this is highly variable depending upon the progress of your research and the time needed to develop into an independent investigator (the primary goal of PhD training).

Both medical school and graduate school are highly demanding and you are expected to perform at a high level and excel in each. Each also requires a very different skill set in order to succeed. Medical schools generally tell you where to be and when. You study the assigned material, take a test, get your scores, and move on to the next set of material. It is a very linear process, heavily based on gaining factual knowledge and being able to apply it. Graduate school is different—you are more independent and expected to progress in your training with little oversight. It is not a one size fits all model like medical school. You are not told where to be, and you generally have to tailor your coursework to your PhD departmental requirements and the particular needs for your proposed project. Hypothesis-driven research requires a significant amount of determination and the ability to think critically and interpret experimental results.

Although there are significant challenges when pursuing a combined degree, there are also significant rewards at the end. Pursuing a MD/PhD makes you more competitive when applying for residency positions. You already have significant research experience and probably at least a couple of publications. You are also more attractive to potential employers after residency and you're likely to have career options that are not available to other physicians: teaching, research, and the pharmaceutical industry.

Despite the difficulties, I can look back on my time pursuing a dual degree and say that it truly represents a time of great personal and professional growth. I am just about to begin residency training in internal medicine so I'm not certain where my career will lead me, but I seem to be gravitating toward staying in an academic center and pursuing clinical research in combination with patient care and teaching. I have no doubt that the pursuit of a dual degree will give me perspective and a great advantage regardless of what I ultimately decide to pursue.

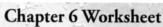

Chapter 6 Worksheet

Dual Degrees

Which dual degree would you be most interested in and why?

How do you think the additional degree would aid in your career as a physician?

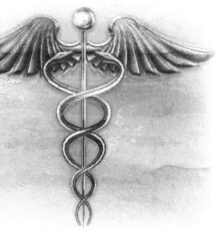

Chapter 7
Medical School Curriculum Preclinical Years

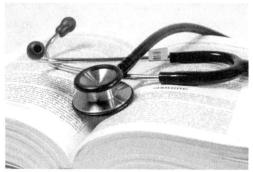

© Gualberto Becerra, 2014. Used under license from Shutterstock, Inc.

The first year to year and a half of medical school have traditionally been known as the basic science years. These tend to be the years where medical students spend a majority of their time in the classroom attending lectures. Although this tradition continues in some schools, the trend is moving away from a large amount of basic science without incorporating clinical content or experience. Some schools have non-traditional styles, and many schools have started to incorporate clinical training, problem based learning, simulation training, team based learning, and other active learning styles into the first two years.

Because students attend medical school to help patients and become a clinician, schools are starting to incorporate exposure to clinical medicine earlier in medical school. Some do this through shadowing experiences, while others have formalized programs allowing students to follow a family or follow patients over time.

Medical simulation is also utilized throughout training. High-fidelity manikins have become much more realistic and can simulate various experiences, such as running a code or delivering a baby. They can also simulate responses to interventions administered, for example, reactions to drugs and procedures. Simulation is used for technical skills as well as communication skills.

In addition to manikins, standardized patients (actors) are used to simulate situations like breaking bad news and resolving patient and family conflict and communication. Standardized patients provide an opportunity for students to practice diagnostic skills with

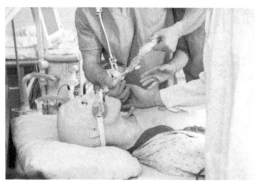

© Tyler Olson, 2014. Used under license from Shutterstock, Inc.

real people. Students may even perform minor, routine procedures on standardized patients followed by feedback from the "patient," faculty members, and fellow students observing the experience.

Team Based Learning is a form of active learning that has caught on in some medical schools. It can be used as an alternative to small group work when there's a large class with minimal faculty. The students are put into groups of seven or so and asked to work together. The session usually consists of both individual and group work. This is a popular approach because it has shown some positive results. For example, Duke University-National University of Singapore Graduate Medical School has decided to adopt this instructional method because of the results it has yielded on standardized exams.

Although new educational techniques are being employed, the majority of schools continue to focus the first two years on basic science topics such as pathophysiology, pharmacology, anatomy, biochemistry, etc. If a student has a solid pre-medical education, the first year of medical school can be a bit less stressful. This is incredibly helpful since the first year is quite an adjustment. Students who seem to adjust more easily to first year commonly state that they had a solid basic science education in either their undergraduate work or in a preparatory masters program.

These topics can be introduced in many organizational ways. Some schools introduce the material within organ systems/blocks and others

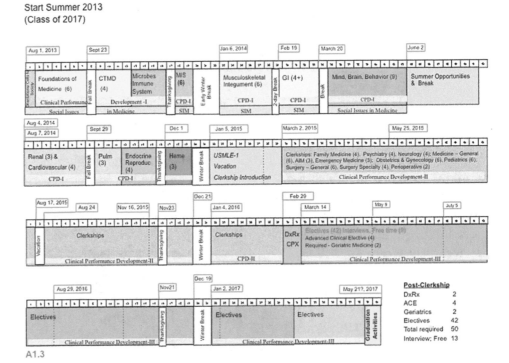

A1.3

introduce them in topic blocks similar to that of a traditional curriculum where subject courses are taken during a semester (like undergraduate school). Other schools introduce the topics through case-based learning, which is popular with students because it is an applied approach that incorporates clinical scenarios and requires critical thinking.

The variety of education methods illustrates that despite the conservative nature of medicine, medical education is constantly evolving. The aforementioned educational methods are currently popular because they have been proven effective, but education will evolve as new methods are utilized, evaluated, and found to be successful. Students who interview for medical school should understand their learning style and the schools' educational methods to ensure they are a fit for their chosen program.

Evolution of educational methods is not the only thing changing in medical school, there are also evolving curriculum organization designs. For example, preclinical years may be shortened to 18 months rather than 2 years. Thus, reviewing each institution's curriculum prior to choosing an institution is very important.

Another interesting trend is the 3 year family medicine curriculum. In order to both encourage students to seek family medicine and to remedy a need for primary care physicians, a couple of schools now offer a 3 year family medicine program. Another benefit to this shortened program is the fact that it also saves these students an extra year of loans/funding (see Texas Tech's curriculum schematic).

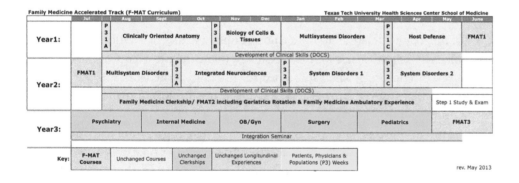

While on the topic of a 3 year curriculum, there is some conversation about shortening medical school in general; this would help reduce the amount of debt accrued and enable physicians to start their careers earlier (http://www.nejm.org/doi/pdf/10.1056/NEJMp1304681). As it is now, many do not start their career (post schooling career) before the age of 30. The schools that currently offer this shortened program often have connections with residencies and place their students into those residencies after graduation.

Grades and Testing

In addition to a variety of educational and teaching methods, there are many assessment methods. Students will be evaluated in traditional and non-traditional ways. There are tests, written and oral presentations, reflection papers, small group evaluation, peer evaluation, etc. Any number of these evaluations can be used while in the first two years. For example:

Communication skills can be evaluated through a standardized patient evaluation; evaluate knowledge of theories through written exams; evaluate application of theories through reflection papers or presentations. Because grades are partial determinates for residency, knowing which type of evaluation method a program predominately uses is helpful.

As though a student is not tested enough, at the end of their preclinical years, they will take the first Step of three USMLE CK Exams (United States Medical Licensing Exam – Clinical Knowledge). It is also important to note that some institutions use traditional letter grades, while others use pass/fail or pass/fail honors. Students often refer to this exam as Step 1 (more information provided in *Chapter 6: Medical School Curriculum Clinical Years*. Much of the first and second year curriculum should prepare the student for this exam; however, many students study review books and review questions in addition to their traditional coursework. The score on this exam is important because it will be part of the application packet sent to residency programs during residency match.

Adjustment

One of the major adjustments from undergraduate school to medical school (note that medical school is also called undergraduate medical education [UME], which can be confusing when shortened to "undergraduate work") is the amount of material that is given for mastery. However, it is important to remember that faculty members knowingly give students more information than they can possibly retain. This process contributes to students developing as adult learners, which includes teaching themselves and understanding what is important to retain.

Due to the volume of information, some students find that their previous way of studying does not work in medical school and they quickly have to adjust their methods. Study groups are formed, tutor or mentor relationships developed, and study buddies are found to maximize retention of material.

Students' self-initiated tactics for studying usually yield positive results, but there are other options as well. Some schools set up peer tutoring or have learning specialists to help students evaluate the effectiveness of their current study style. Something to keep in mind is that once a student is admitted to medical school, the program is then invested in that student and wants that student to do well.

Academic adjustment is not the only thing students have to work with. They also have to adjust to the new lifestyle of putting medicine first. Some students have had to miss weddings and family vacations due to studies. If a student ever finds they are overwhelmed emotionally, schools offer emotional support through their Student Affairs office and even counseling. So, although it may seem like a "dog eat dog" world with the fast-paced curriculum and tests, there is a structure in place to help students be successful. Administration and faculty have a vested interest in students' success and will help in every way they can. If a student needs something within reason, most likely Student Affairs will work to ensure it happens.

Additional Curricular Topics

Because medicine is an art, mastery of basic science topics is not sufficient. Students must also master social science topics, clinical skills, evidence based medicine, and other topics that are deemed necessary for becoming a clinician. Medical ethics as a topic is included in most curriculums. Often, these topics are addressed through small group interaction with case scenarios. The scenarios are designed to make students think about how they would respond in certain situations. A common scenario is built around a child who is hospitalized and happens to be Jehovah's Witness. As a Jehovah's Witness, blood transfusions are not permitted. This child needs a transfusion desperately. As the physician, what do you do? This question is posed with follow-up questions for group discussion.

The case below is another example that was used in previous curriculum. First students were given a lecture around laws and ethics of sexual harassment. Following the lecture, they met in groups to discuss a handful of cases.

Sample Case

Jill is a 3rd year medical student who is interested in surgery. She has great rapport with the director of the surgical clerkship and respects his vision and ideas about where the department is going. However, Jill is becoming a bit concerned about the conversations in the OR. While assisting on a case, Jill quietly retracts and is subjected to a conversation that two residents are having about their weekend. These conversations include escapades with the opposite sex. One of the residents begins to discuss his "conquest" in detail. Although Jill is quite uncomfortable, she decides to ignore it as a one-time event. Unfortunately, the very next day in the OR these types of conversations are repeated. Jill feels incredibly uncomfortable, but does not want to say anything to the clerkship director who she respects.

Is this sexual harassment? If so, how would you classify it?

Why would Jill not want to tell her director?

What are the issues that Jill might face if she does or does not tell someone about this situation?

Evidence Based Medicine

Another topic that is becoming more prevalent in the first and second year is evidence based medicine. This curriculum usually includes some public health, biostatistics, and basic research evaluation tools. This surge in curriculum has come from the larger picture and push to incorporate evidence into practice as well as critically appraise evidence by looking at the methods used within the research and questioning conclusions that are drawn with a critical eye. This skill is important because of the amount of research being published that physicians must sift through and evaluate to make educated decisions.

Scholarship

Some medical schools require a scholarship component to their medical degree, while others simply offer it as an option. Scholarship can include things like the study of public health, public policy, or translational research. These are just a few options. Some schools have a community presence and use full immersion into a community project as a scholarship endeavor. These projects serve many purposes. Each institution has a set of goals for their scholarly program and they vary from encouraging scientific inquiry to encouraging lifelong learning. If the school requires the scholarship concentration, then placement into a program of study will be more seamless and organized. However, it may also be a bit more limited or rigid, as the educational goals may require specific areas of study. Required or not, most programs will ensure students have faculty advisors to help them through the process, acting much like a mentor. The addition of a scholarship program to the curriculum is important to note because it comes with a whole new set of questions. For example: How much curricular time is dedicated to this program/project? How much support is a student given to complete their project? Will the student have autonomy in choosing the scholarly topic? These are all potential interview questions for the medical student applicant to ask of the schools requiring a scholarly concentration or scholarly program (provided the answers are not listed on the program's website). Below Stanford's curriculum schematic demonstrates the addition of a scholarly concentration.

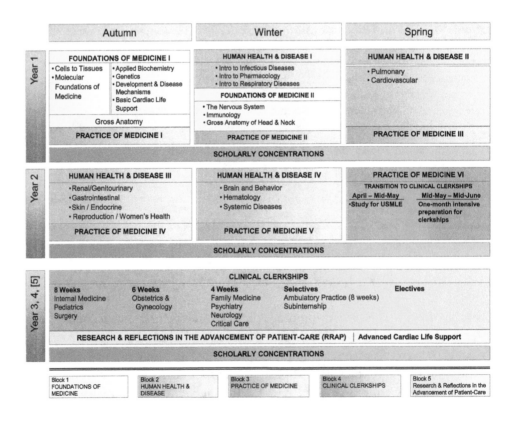

Scheduling

The amount of information that is thrown at a student requires excessive study. So much study that medical school becomes a full-time job. During the day, students attend lectures and other learning opportunities and night is dedicated to studying and preparing for tests.

Just like undergraduate education, medical school also has its fair share of extracurricular activities. These activities are to be fit into the already busy schedule of a student. Some of the following are examples of the many opportunities that exist for students: research participation, student government and organization positions, and intramural sports. None of these activities are required, however, students participate for a multitude of reasons (future marketability during residency match, facilitating friendships or mentorships, gaining leadership experience, or just to simply satisfy an inherent interest).

Once a student has made it to the clinical years, they feel a renewed sense of excitement because they will have much more exposure to patients. This renewed excitement and hope is soon met with the reality of clinical demands in third year.

Reflection from a 2nd Year Medical Student

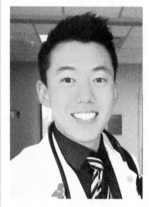

By Min "Sam" Han
Texas A&M Health Science Center College of
Medicine, Class of 2015

As my teammates and I grabbed the metal handles to open our "tank," I couldn't help but have a flashback of the past few days of class. We had learned about the coronary arteries and the different branches that supplied the heart. We learned that a normal ejection fraction of the heart was about 55%, and that the contraction force of this small organ enabled blood to be shunted to our entire body. And here I was scalpel in hand, about to cut into the thorax. In a few short minutes, I would be holding a human heart in my hand.

The first year of medical school was quite fascinating. While trying to hold back my excitement each and every day, I was running in and out between anatomy, histology, and other basic science courses and anatomy and histology labs. For example, in the morning, our class would learn about the different changes in cell types lining our upper and lower respiratory system. In the afternoon, we would go into the lab and actually observe the changes in the respiratory epithelium ourselves. The greatest experience of first year was without a doubt our anatomy lab course. From holding the heart in my hands, opening up the skull to visualize the brain, visualizing the 34 different muscles moving our fingers, and cleaning up stool from the colon, there was never a dull moment.

During our second year, we learned the pharmacology, pathology, and physiology of all the different organ systems. This was our year to really focus and learn as much as possible. Part I of our medical board exam was looming in the horizon, and we knew it would be one of the most important exams in our lives. Many afternoons were filled with doing practice questions, flipping through flash cards, and reading different pathology books. I didn't quite expect how much this focused studying would also help in providing quality care for my future patients.

continued

Reflection from a 2nd Year Medical Student *(continued)*

Hundreds of patients had lined up at a local church in Lima, Peru. Several of our classmates had decided to serve with a few of our teaching physicians in Lima during spring break. I remember one particular patient encounter. "I'm having severe pain in my shoulders, and I can't raise my arms. I need to work in my textile factory to provide for my family, but I won't be able to work if this pain won't go away. It's been going on for months, and I can't work." The older woman looked at me intensely with eyes that were filled with fear but with a glimpse of hope. A few minutes after injecting a steroid shot and giving her some medications, tears started streaming down her eyes. She was able to move her arms up and down without feeling any pain. She ran up to us after the clinic was over with bags of fruits and bracelets she had bought from the local market. Right then, I realized that the hours of studying behind a desk, learning about all the different actions of muscles, the mechanisms of drugs, and the physiology of our organ systems had surely paid off. I was now ready for my clinical years.

Chapter 7 Worksheet

Preclinical Curriculum

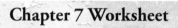

List your top two medical schools from the Chapter 2 Worksheet:

1)

2)

What are the main curricular components of the preclinical years for each school?

1)

2)

Differences	**Similarities**

What is important to you in medical school regarding curriculum (type of learning, experiences, etc.)?

Which school matches your interests more and why?

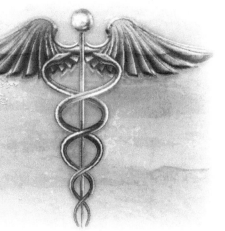

Chapter 8
Medical School Curriculum Clinical Years

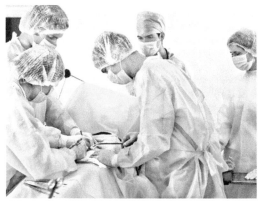

© Poznyakov, 2014. Used under license from Shutterstock, Inc.

Following the preclinical education, most medical schools include 2–2.5 years of clinical training. This is the time when medical students have the opportunity to concentrate their learning within the clinical setting, seeing patients, and working alongside residents, fellows, and staff physicians (also known as attending physicians; "attending" for short). Each aspect of the clinical years is described in more detail below.

Core Rotations

Many medical schools offer the opportunity for students to interact with patients and physicians during their preclinical years of medical school, however the bulk of that training will begin in the clinical years. There may be some variation in specialty exposure, but most medical schools provide exposure to the core areas of medicine needed for a strong foundation of knowledge, not only for later training (residency) but also for board exam preparation (described below under *4th Year of Medical School*).

Traditional Model

The first part of the clinical years exposes medical students to various fields of medicine for the basic foundation mentioned above and to help students solidify their decision about future practice. Medical school curricula follow varying structures for the clinical years. One of the traditional formats is to complete the core rotations consecutively followed by elective rotations. Figure 8.1 depicts the traditional model for core rotations. The order that students rotate through these and the time spent in each field will vary.

Figure 8-1.

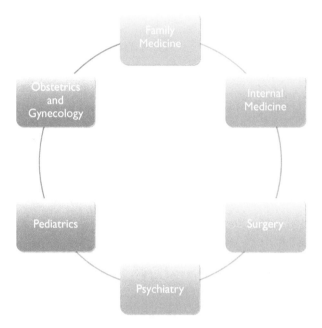

Some schools may add time for rotating through other areas such as radiology, anesthesiology, emergency medicine, and other specialties. Students often have the opportunity for exposure to the subspecialties within these areas when on the rotation (e.g., orthopedic surgery during surgery rotation). However, exposure to other fields or in subspecialty areas is often reserved for the 4th year. Some structures will allow for exposure to specialty/subspecialty exposure interspersed between the core-rotations, particularly if more time is allotted to the clinical training prior to the 4th year.

Longitudinal/Integrated Model

Some schools utilize a longitudinal integrated clinical training module, during which these core rotations are taken concurrently. The model that Texas A&M

Figure 8-2.

Student:			Mentor:			
Week 1	**Monday**	**Tuesday**	**Wednesday**	**Thursday**	**Friday**	**Weekend**
7:00am	Hospital Rounds	Hospital Rounds	Hospital Rounds	Hospital Rounds	Hospital Rounds	Hosp Rds
	↓	↓	↓	↓	↓	
8:30am	Family Medicine Clinic	Opportunity Time	Surgery Clinic & OR	Opportunity Time	PEDS Clinic	Call 8am-11pm (On Call in ER, Surgery, L&D) (8 Hr. Shift)
Noon						
1:00pm		Opportunity Time		Opportunity Time	AIM Time	
5:00pm		AIM Teach				
6:00pm	Weekday Call		Weekday call 6pm-11pm (On Call in ER, Surgery, L&D)			
Week 2	**Monday**	**Tuesday**	**Wednesday**	**Thursday**	**Friday**	**Weekend**
7:00am	Hospital Rounds	Hospital Rounds	Hospital Rounds	Hospital Rounds	Hospital Rounds	Hosp Rds
	↓	↓	↓	↓	↓	
8:30am	OB/Gyn Clinic & OR	Opportunity Time	Psychiatry	Opportunity Time	Internal Medicine Clinic	Call 8am-11pm (On Call in ER, Surgery, L&D) (8 Hr. Shift)
Noon						
1:00pm		Opportunity Time		Opportunity Time	AIM Time	
5:00pm			Opportunity Time	Opportunity Time		
		AIM Teach				
6:00pm	Weekday Call		Weekday call 6pm-11pm (On Call in ER, Surgery, L&D)			

College of Medicine uses is shown in Figure 8.2. In this structure, students are able to follow patients and illness or condition evolution over a longer period of time.

Schedule

As previously mentioned, the schedule for each of the core rotations may vary. Coming from the classroom/study setting of the preclinical years, the clinical schedule will feel like a work schedule. Some rotations may have the student reporting to the hospital at 5 a.m. (or even earlier) to prepare for surgery, while others may include working long hours in a clinic. Much of this will depend not only on the rotation, but also the setting and specialty. Students may be rotating in a hospital or in a clinic, and each setting will have different business hours. Depending on the rotation, students may also be expected to take night call. That means they would carry a pager and respond as necessary. For example, a student who is on a surgical trauma service may be assigned night call to ensure he/she had as much exposure to the cases as possible.

Professionalism

In the preclinical years, medical students are often taught about professionalism as part of their curriculum, however in clinical years, they will be expected to put what they have learned into practice. The preclinical schedule may have allowed for the student to have flexibility in terms of which classes they attended in person or what they wore when they went to class. Other than the extensive workload, it may feel a bit like an extension of the undergraduate years. However, in the clinical years, students are now interacting with actual patients in a professional setting, therefore the expectations are altered to that of the culture of clinical medicine. Anything that is true for a paid professional job is true for this environment. They must not be late in reporting since they are working directly with patients and are also working in a team of health care professionals who rely on one another. They must also wear appropriate attire for the setting. Most rotations will require that students wear professional clothes. This does not mean the suit the student wore when he/she interviewed for medical school, but slacks and a button up shirt for men and slacks/skirt, and a blouse for women. Students' behavior must always be professional as well. Some think professional behavior is simply understood, however, students need to make conscious effort to always maintain professional behavior. Additionally, students should avoid inappropriate relationships, conversations, and posts on social media.

Studying

Being out of the classroom does not mean the end of studying. There will be many topics students will encounter every day that they do not know and will need to spend time reading about (e.g., diseases, treatment, and research). Students also spend time improving their history and physical exam skills. Because physicians' time is limited, it is important that this time is spent creating an efficient and effective way of interacting with the patient.

There is also time spent learning about deducing a diagnosis and creating a treatment plan. These activities are done in a non-threatening learning environment. Students also spend time learning about disease prognosis, both what is in the literature and what the physicians they are working with have experienced. It is important each case is attended to because they may be quizzed about it later or expected to report back to the team. Students will also be reading about their patients' conditions, which is important in order to follow along with what is being discussed.

Following each rotation, there will be an exam called a shelf exam. These exams are provided by the National Board of Medical Examiners (NBME), which assess knowledge in each of the areas. Each rotation may factor in different items for grading the rotations in addition to the shelf exam, including quizzes, attending physicians' evaluations, and exams. Each rotation's grade may vary on how much weight is given to each aspect.

Preparing for 4th Year

As students go through their core rotations, they are beginning to narrow down the fields of medicine that interest them. Some come to medical school with previous exposure and have a good idea of what kind of physician they want to be, while others will determine that by going through the rotations. During the 3rd year, students will begin planning their 4th year rotations. Although there are some requirements within the 4th year, most of this year is meant to plan rotations in the area of interest and locations where students are considering applying for residency.

Planning for 4th year will require another application process for away rotations. In the past, students had to submit applications to each individual away rotation. However, with the creation and implementation of VSAS, Visiting Student Application Service, students are able to complete one online application and send that application out to any away rotations that participate in the VSAS system. All LCME accredited programs utilize this program as do some participating schools accredited by COCA, Commission on Osteopathic College Accreditation (https://www.aamc.org/students/medstudents/vsas?about_vsas/272382/participatingosteopathicmedicalcolleges.html).

4th Year of Medical School

The fourth year of medical school is often the "light at the end of the tunnel" year for medical students. They have worked long and hard hours over the past three years and are looking forward to their scheduled rotations in the areas that interest them. The scheduled rotations are also known as elective rotations and sometimes called "try out" rotations. The amount of elective time or away rotations available for the student depends on the curriculum time dedicated to required material during 4th year. Thus, this is an important aspect to note when interviewing for medical school. Some schools require more advanced rotations during the 4th year (e.g., an AI, also known as an acting internship; this rotation gives students an opportunity to present themselves as an intern and take on extra responsibility that will hopefully prepare them for their internship year. Another example is an intensive care unit rotation. Students are asked to do this rotation during their fourth year because that is when they have the foundational information to better grasp the nuances of critical patients.).

If electives are allowed outside of the medical school's affiliated hospitals/clinics, students should plan a rotation at a site where they are interested in completing residency. This gives them time to explore the program and get to know the faculty and residents there; hence, the name "try out rotation." This is a wonderful and stressful time because students are doing what they want to do, but they are also trying to make a good impression for the future residency match and to gain an interview. These rotations are quite important because some programs favor students who spend time at their institution.

USMLE Step 2 and COMLEX Level 2 Exams

During 4th year, students will take the Step II of the United States Medical Licensing Examination (USMLE) for MD students or the Level 2 Comprehensive Osteopathic Medical Licensing Examination (COMLEX) for DO students. DO students who plan to enter the MD match (AMA) will take both exams. The USMLE Step 2 is composed of two parts: Step 2 Clinical Knowledge (CK) and Step 2 Clinical Skills (CS). The COMLEX Level 2 includes: Level 2 Cognitive Evaluation (CE) and Level 2 Performance Evaluation (PE).

- USMLE Step 2 Clinical Knowledge: This exam assesses the student's ability to apply medical knowledge, skills, and understanding of clinical science to providing patient care.
- USMLE Step 2 Clinical Skills: This exam assesses the student's mastery of clinical skills tested in a standardized patient[*] setting.
- COMLEX Level 2 Cognitive Evaluation: Students must demonstrate knowledge of clinical concepts and medical decision-making.
- COMLEX Level 2 Performance Evaluation: Similar to the USMLE Step 2 CS, students are evaluated on their clinical skills using standardized patients.

---

[*]Standardized patients are trained actors who act out symptoms and use a scripted dialogue.

Reflections from a 4th Year Medical Student

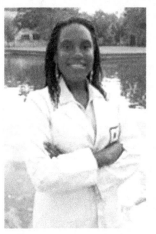

By Charity Idowu, MD
Texas A&M Health Science Center
   College of Medicine, Class of 2013
Residency: Internal Medicine – Pediatrics, University of
   Rochester, Strong Memorial Hospital, Rochester, NY

The last two years of medical school are a time when everything that you have learned during the first two years starts coming together. You begin your clinical rotations and realize that the art of medicine is more than just knowing facts but about knowing how these facts relate to real human beings. As a third and fourth year medical student, you are considered a member of the care team whose input truly matters. Your studying is more directed towards the diagnosis and treatment of actual patients that you see day to day. You begin to take into consideration how a patient's social situation is affected by their condition and the clinical decisions that your team makes. One aspect that I had to adjust to was the fact that there is not always a clear diagnosis for every patient as you normally see written in textbooks. However, this aspect is what makes the field of medicine such an interesting art that can never grow old. What I felt prepared me the most for residency as well as the practice of searching the literature and coming up with my own plan for each of my patients before asking for input from staff physicians or residents. I always asked myself, "What would I do for this patient if I was the only one here to make a decision?" I realized that the clinical years of medical school are not about always having the right answers but are about learning how to think critically and coming up with ideas that make sense clinically.

List your top two medical schools from the Chapter 2 Worksheet:

1)

2)

What are the main curricular components of the clinical years for each school?

1)

2)

Differences	Similarities

Which school matches your interests more and why?

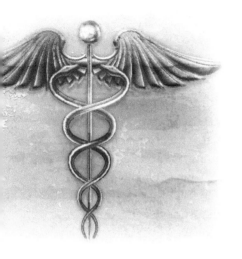

Chapter 9
Residency Application Process

Successful **Residency Application (ERAS)** should lead to:	An Interview offer. **Successful Interviews** should lead to:	**Match**

During the summer and early fall of the final year of medical school; students are preparing to apply for residency programs in their chosen field. Just like applying to medical school, students will submit a lengthy application with supporting documents for residency programs to consider for an interview and ultimately a residency spot.

Residency Application

The residency application is a student's opportunity to put their best foot forward and to hopefully convince their chosen residency programs that they are a "fit" for that program. The application will only get the student in the door for the interview. Often students are quite determined to get into specific programs without considering if the program is actually a fit for him or her. For example, a student may be completely set on attending a program on the east coast, but every program that the student has chosen focuses heavily on research and the student has no interest in research. This is a mismatch in goals and the program will most likely see this and not offer the student an interview. Alternatively, they may become aware of the mismatch during the interview and ultimately not offer the student a spot for residency. Matching to a program is somewhat parallel to a relationship. Everyone has wanted to date someone who didn't want to date him or her back. It is not that either party is not good enough for the other but instead that something doesn't fit or match. Although match initially seems like a term used for Electronic Residency Application Service (ERAS) purposes, if thought about, it is an excellent word to describe what is being done, finding a match or fit between the candidate and the program.

In order to ensure a positive match outcome, the student will want to research programs and attempt to apply to programs for which he/she will best fit. Additionally, the student will want to use this research while preparing their application, and preparing for the interview.

Application Components

Letters of Recommendation

Although this is a required component to the application, the student does have some liberty in deciding who will best represent him/her to their chosen specialty. This component of the residency application will require the student to go out and ask faculty to write a letter of recommendation on their behalf. Thus, it is important that the student has given the faculty member an opportunity to see their abilities and personality throughout their time together. It is helpful if the letters are personal. Most of all, the entire letter should have only the highest recommendation. Statements such as "I highly recommend. . ." or "I recommend this person without reservation. . ." will make the most positive impact. Statements with less support will send up red flags.

Students may also obtain additional letters from faculty and submit them to specific schools. For example, if a student plans to apply to Cleveland Clinic's Internal Medicine Program and has worked with a graduate of that program, they may want to ask for a letter from that graduate to add to their Cleveland Clinic application. Thus, students do not have to submit the same letters to every program. In theory, a student could upload several letters but select which program receives which letter. The hope is that having a letter from an alumnus of the program for which the student is applying is an added value.

The letters are very important to faculty selecting students for residency. Some programs find them more helpful than the personal statement or Dean's Letter (described below). Some program directors believe the personal statement is less authentic than the letters of recommendation and that the Dean's Letter is not as informative or personal. With this is in mind, the onus is on the student to find faculty who will represent them well within the letter. Students will want to choose faculty who have seen them at their best and know them in a positive way. The letter should leave no doubt for a future employer. One way to ensure this is to have an honest conversation with letter writers. Ask the letter writer if he/she feels comfortable writing a positive letter of recommendation. If the answer does not sound confident, then the student should reconsider the choice. Another way to ensure a positive letter is to have a Curriculum Vitae and personal statement ready when requesting the letter. Some faculty will request a meeting to receive additional personal information to be included in the personal statement. This background information will help the faculty member write something a bit more personal. Finally, it is also important to note that not all specialties adhere to the same requirements. For example, Emergency Medicine uses a Standardized Letter of Evaluation (SLOE), which is more of an evaluative tool rather than a letter of recommendation. Know your specialty and what the specialty and what your specialty requires.

Medical Student Performance Evaluation (MSPE) (Also known as: Dean's Letter)

MSPE sometimes referred to as the Dean's Letter is another required component that is traditionally written by the Student Affairs Dean. Much of this letter is a compilation of the required rotations' evaluation summaries. Therefore, it is imperative that the student performs well both academically and professionally. The student affairs dean will sift through 4 years of evaluations and compile them in sequential order to make one letter from the medical school. This letter is not meant to be a letter of recommendation, but instead a letter to summarize the student's performance as compared to their peers. In the past, this letter was posted later in the application/interview season and many programs had already offered interviews without having seen the Dean's Letter. In order to make the letter a more important part of the application and make the letter available to programs for their decision-making process, the AAMC pushed up the due date.

Personal Statement

Students will have to once again write a personal statement, however, this time the question will be which specialty was chosen and why. Students often pull up their old personal statement from the medical school application and try to salvage some of that content. However, those statements often do not contain the content or insight that a program seeks. The statement should be written with the new goals of residency in mind. Personal statements should be about a page in length. Other questions to consider while writing a personal statement along with sample excerpts are listed below:

Why have you chosen your specialty?
How did you make your choice?
What about the specialty appeals to you?
When did you realize that you wanted to be (chosen specialty)...?

> **Example:**
>
> While rotating through the emergency department, I quickly noticed that the diversity and pace of the Emergency Department not only excited me, but also reminded me of my original purpose in medicine, helping people in acute situations.

The answers to these questions should help the program understand the student's reasons for wanting to enter their specialty. Faculty members are looking for authentic answers that potentially match up with their ideal candidate.

> What makes you unique?
> What will you bring to the program?
> What makes you a good fit?

> **Example:**
>
> Growing up in south Texas has given me a unique perspective and love for the Hispanic culture. Serving this population would be an amazing honor and your program would afford...

The answers to these questions should help faculty get to know the student and help the student stand out from other applicants. If the statement is interesting enough, it could help the student receive an interview and may be a topic of conversation during the interview.

> What are you looking for in a program?
> Research opportunities?
> Teaching opportunities?
> Exposure to types of procedures or...??

> **Example:**
>
> As a family physician, exposure to a vast array of patients, diagnoses is imparative...
>
> Or
>
> Participating in and contributing to research in medicine has been extraordinarily rewarding for me. Thus, I hope to continue...

The answers to these questions should help the program see if the student is a fit for the program. Is the student looking for something the program can give them? Are the student's needs and wants in line with the program?

> What are your career goals?

> **Example:**
>
> Following residency, I plan to pursue a fellowship and ultimately hope to work in a level 1 academic center...

The answers to this question should also help the program decide about fit.

Overall, answers to these questions should coincide with what the program is looking for. For example, if the student says that he/she is interested in research, the programs should also be interested in research.

A common denominator with personal statements that left a lasting positive impression was that they were authentic and vulnerable. Students opened up and shared something that stood out from others. Another common denominator was a lack of mistakes. Students who had multiple people read their statements for grammatical, syntax, and spelling issues also had stronger statements. Finally, the statements that stood out above all were those that did all of the above and included at least three drafts.

The following are some helpful hints for writing a personal statement. When beginning, consider the previously listed questions (what specialty and why) and write an outline to help ensure everything is addressed. Get to the point early on. It is important that the statement catches the attention of the reader quickly as many program faculty members do not have time to read the whole application. Students will often find that the people interviewing them have not read their personal statement, thus getting to the point quickly is more likely to result in a statement being read. The statement should also be an easy and straightforward read. Students should not forget the rules of basic writing composition such as having a thesis statement for each paragraph followed by supporting sentences and then having a summary statement. These helpful hints as well as the topics to avoid (listed next) should ensure that a student is not ruled out based on issues within the personal statement.

Just as there are some "dos"; there are also some "don'ts". Students should avoid any controversial topics such as religion, politics, or anything that could strike up a heated conversation. No assumptions should be made about the person reading the statement or their views, as being wrong could jeopardize being offered an interview. Although vulnerability was mentioned previously as a positive, over-sharing or getting too personal can be seen as instability or negative. Students should also strike a balance between modesty and arrogance. Some programs look for too many "I" statements as a sign of arrogance, or self-centeredness. Finally, the students should be sure the statement sounds like and represents them well, therefore language or vocabulary that does not suit them should be avoided. The statement should reflect the applicant not how well the applicant can use the thesaurus.

Curriculum Vitae (CV)

The CV is a running record of things a student has done and hopefully has been continually added to since first applying to medical school. The CV is a promotional document and has some steadfast rules. Some of these rules include:

- Sections and events should be listed in reverse chronological order.
- The language within the section should coincide with the date listed. For example, if the event was in the past, then the descriptors should

be in the past as well. If the position is listed as present, then the language should be present.

- Two things that are commonly seen on CVs that are no longer standard or necessary are titling the CV "Curriculum Vitae" and listing references at the bottom. Both were previously done, but are no longer considered necessary.

- Concise language and avoiding redundancy is another way to conserve room and keep your reviewer intrigued. If a student has several experiences within similar fields, they will want to avoid listing the same descriptors. Also, try and keep the descriptors to three lines.

- Students will also want to keep their listings relevant and current. It is okay to list older experiences as long as they are relevant to the student's future or they serve as positive promotion of the student. It is also okay to leave recent experiences off if they are deemed irrelevant. For example, if a student has spent time working at a tax preparation company to make some extra money, but does not see that it is relevant to their future career, then it is okay to eliminate that listing.

- One of the last steadfast rules is consistency in all of the following:
  - Formatting of the listings, how dates of service are listed, and how punctuation is used.
  - If periods are used after position descriptors, then be sure that they are used after every descriptor.
  - If the position title is italicized for one listing, ensure all other listings have italicized titles.
  - If the date is listed as a month and year, then all dates throughout need to be listed as such.
  - Also, the location of each piece within the section listing should be consistent. If the dates are listed to left, then all dates need to be listed to the left, etc.

These details will help the CV look clean and easy to read as it will enable the reader to find listing information in a quick fashion.

With the steadfast rules aside, it is important to note that order of section listings and title of section listings are not always going to be the same across the board. Students will want to list things that are most important to them first as well as using headings that promote them best. The only heading that should be included on all CVs is "Education". The rest are relative to that student's experience. For example, a student will not want an awards section heading if they have no awards of significance to report. However, the CV created within the ERAS system does include certain descriptors. The easiest way to prepare for the ERAS CV is to ensure the CV is up to date and then use that information to create the document within ERAS.

USMLE and Grades

As always, grades are an important part of the application process. Although all grades will be reviewed, many programs will look specifically at rotation grades that are relevant to the student's future specialty. If a student is applying to internal medicine, then the program will want to know how the student did on their internal medicine rotation. Other specialties may find anatomy grades to be helpful.

Another score that is heavily weighed by many programs is the step score. Some students will have USMLE scores, others will have COMLEX scores, and some will have both. Often osteopathic medical students will take both step exams to ensure that they have scores that are easily understood and comparable for allopathic GME programs. At the time of application, some students will have taken steps 1 and 2 and some will only have the first step to report. If a student's step 1 score was not at the level he/she wanted then he/she will want to work hard to ensure their step 2 score is an improvement and to have those scores available in time for the application process.

Interviewing

Interviews for residency will begin in the fall and typically end sometime in late winter. Students should be prepared to travel around the country for interviews.

Once a student has been asked to interview, the research about that program should begin. This will allow the student to tailor their answers and questions to ensure they appear prepared and educated about each program. Students should be prepared for different styles of interviews and for different types of interview questions. Interviews can range from one interviewer, to panel interviews to multiple interviewees being interviewed at one time. Regardless of the interview style, a student can expect to have a full day of interviewing activities and touring the program site. Some programs will host a pre-interview dinner the night before the interview day. This interview dinner gives students an opportunity to ask informal questions like what a regular week is like as a resident or what kind of procedures are most common within the practice there. The student must keep in mind that the environment feels informal, but it is still an interview. Thus, the tone should always be positive and professional. In other words, students should not say anything that they would not say in a formal interview.

Students should be mindful the interview begins when a student first makes contact with the program. Program coordinators, administrators, and anyone who speaks with the student may be solicited for feedback on the applicant. If the student is participating in an away rotation, they are essentially on an interview rotation. Social media can also enter into the screening process for an applicant. Some programs google all the applicants they interview. With this in mind, students should manage their online profile and be very discrete, as online professionalism has become as important as in person professionalism. A small lapse in judgment such as an inappropriate comment or photo could cost a student a residency interview or residency spot.

On the actual interview day, students can expect to meet with several members of administration and should be prepared to answer questions about their application (anything within the application is fair for questioning). They should also expect to answer some basic common questions such as:

Tell me about yourself

The answer to this question should be prepared so that it is succinct and has a beginning, middle, and ending.

> Information to include:
> Where the student was born and reared
> Where the student went to undergrad
> A few interesting facts
> Where the student went to medical school
> How the student decided what they wanted to do

Here's an example of how an answer could begin:

> I was born in Houston, Texas and attended Rice University for undergraduate work. While in undergrad, I volunteered at the local free clinic and participated in two international mission trips. These experiences solidified my interest in working with medically underserved populations, and led me to apply to medical school. I was accepted at the University of Texas HSC San Antonio where I continue to work with underserved populations and participate in medical missions. These experiences have encouraged me to specialize in ophthalmology, as....

Why do you want to be a ___?

Here interviewers are looking for a genuine answer that is not self-serving.

What are your future goals?

Here interviewers are looking for a fit for their program, so the student will want to ensure their answer coincides with the programs goals. If the student mentions that they are extremely interested in academia and the program has no interest in academia then it will be assumed that the student is not a fit for the program.

Why are you interested in our program?

This is an opportunity for the student to demonstrate their knowledge of the program.

Why should we choose you?

This is the student's opportunity to share their positive attributes and what they can contribute to the program.

Do you have any questions for us?

The answer to this question is always yes. Students should prepare questions in advance and write down questions as they think of them during the interview.

These are just some of the common questions asked within the interview, however, some interviews may be much more informal resulting in a conversation.

Another type of question to consider is the behavioral interview question. It is believed that industrial and organizational psychologists developed this type of questioning in the 1970s. The theory behind its development was that *past behavior is the best predictor of future behavior*, thus having a candidate report about what they have done versus what they would do is a better predictor of performance. For example, an interviewer might say, "What would you do if you were working with a colleague and witnessed something unethical?" The candidate is sure to tell the interviewer that he/she would most certainly report the offence or handle the situation in the most ideal way. In this example, the response is about how great the applicant can be, instead of how great the applicant will be. So, instead, an interviewer asks the candidate "Tell me about a time that you witnessed something you thought was unethical," this requires the applicant to recall an actual situation and disclose how the situation was handled. This type of answer is more likely to be a predictor of how the candidate would handle a future situation than that of a "what would you do" question as the "what would you do" question is set up for an ideal situation without complications or external variables, where there are no consequences for doing the right thing, and where the applicant will be supported in taking any action.

Just as there are formulas to other questions, there is also a formula to this type of question. It is important that applicants fully answer the question in an organized and succinct way. The most common method utilized to ensure a thorough answer is the STAR method.

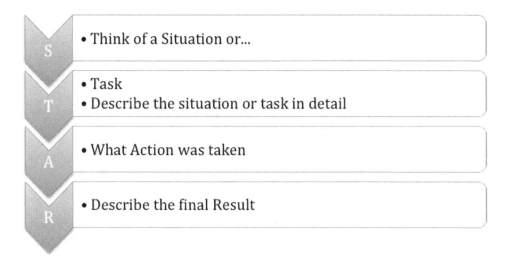

- **S** • Think of a Situation or…
- **T** • Task
  • Describe the situation or task in detail
- **A** • What Action was taken
- **R** • Describe the final Result

This should be done in a succinct manor and sound much like a story. Following is an example using this technique:

> *Tell me about a time that you witnessed something you thought was unethical*
> S/T
> While on my Acting Internship with a colleague, I noticed that he would often leave after the first surgery of the day. We are not supposed to leave

until we have checked out with the chief resident. Because the surgeons are so busy, they were not asking for him, so our supervising resident did not address or notice the issue.

A

This left me with the ethical dilemma of whether to say anything or just do my job. After careful consideration, I decided to speak with my colleague and request that he follow the rules.

R

Fortunately, he understood that his absence was putting me in a bad situation and reflecting poorly on our school, not to mention potentially ruining the autonomy we have for future students. He agreed to follow proper protocol and complete the check-out process in the future.

Beginning in 2018, Emergency Medicine will require a video recorded behavioral interview (Standardized Video Interview). The interview receives a standardized score to be reported in the objective area of the application.

Most people have experienced the situation where they thought they answered a question after rambling for a while and then had to ask their interviewer, "Did I answer your question?" or "Is that what you wanted?" Instead of being unsure, it is better to formulate a great answer with a proven formula.

The last part of the interview is often thought of as a closing, but instead should be thought of as a thank you note. Students should prepare a note that is personal to that program and is timely. This note can also include anything you forgot, but wanted to say in the interview. It is a great way to remind the program about your interest and let them know how thankful you are that they took time to meet with you. This note should be sent at the student's earliest convenience for multiple reasons. One, writing the thank you note is easier when the experience is fresh in mind and two, the note should come promptly after the interview to ensure the program receives it before any ranking decisions are made.

See information on the medical school interview for additional information on how to dress and prepare for the interview day.

Additional Interview Offer Information

Something of note is that some programs do give interviews to students who rotate at their site as a courtesy. This does not always mean that they believe the student to be a good fit for the program, but may simply be a courtesy for rotating at the institution. If a student does not receive an interview offer after participating in an away rotation at an institution, then the faculty members have most likely decided that the student is not a fit for their program.

How to be Competitive

Being a competitive applicant is important and often students find themselves scrambling to build their CVs in the latter part of medical school. Instead, students should be involved throughout their medical school years. Being involved can include an array of activities and leadership roles. This involvement will demonstrate that the student is motivated and has experience in certain areas that may be of interest to particular specialties.

Each medical school has programs that allow students to actively lead or participate. Most schools will also have clinical activities, mission trips, student government, and research opportunities. These activities demonstrate different strengths and characteristics and should be sought to ensure growth and external education for future roles. Different residency programs will look for different types of involvement so knowing what the program values is important and will help make a strong and competitive CV and application.

Although this all sounds incredibly daunting, students should remember that their institutions want them to be successful so there are guidelines and faculty in place to help them through the process. Faculty advisors and student affairs deans will typically help students in deciding how many and which residency programs to apply to. These faculty members are seasoned in the process and know what will most likely end in success for the student.

Residency Match

The national residency match for MD students occurs the third Friday of March every year. As mentioned before, students will submit their application through ERAS. The National Residency Matching Program (NRMP) is the organization that handles the actual match to residency. Students and residency program directors will submit their rank lists through NRMP. The NRMP system then matches the student with the program. The Monday prior to the Friday match, students will learn if they have matched to a residency. If they have not, they will need to participate in the Supplemental Offer and Acceptance Program (SOAP), which works to match students to unfilled residency spots. Most students will find a spot during SOAP. But, if a student finds himself or herself without a residency spot after SOAP, there are alternative options (i.e., research year). Friday, students will receive the notification of where they matched. This match is a contract and once it is revealed, the student is promised to that institution for the duration of residency. Many schools participate in Match Day celebrations where all students find out where they matched together.

There are some programs that match students outside of the national residency match including ophthalmology and neurology. The military residency match also occurs outside of the national match and completes their match in December.

If DO students elect not to participate in the NRMP match, they will participate in matching to a DO residency through the AOA NMS. The AOA match process occurs in February of every year. DO students will need to determine if they want to go through the AOA match process because if matched to an AOA residency program their status will be communicated to NRMP and they will be withdrawn from the NRMP match process. https://natmatch .com/aoairp/aboutoverview.html#withdrawing

However, there are some significant, positive changes coming to this process. The ACGME will soon begin accrediting AOA residencies thereby including them in the NRMP match. In time, there may no longer be a separate process for applying to Graduate Medical Education spots. More information can be found in *Chapter 5: Osteopathic Medicine and Allopathic Medicine.*

Each step of the process has an effect on the next: A successful residency application within the ERAS should result in interview offers; successful interviews should result in match. Once the student receives an interview, it is an indication that the program has decided the student could be a fit based on the information provided within the application. The next step in the process is the interview. The student will want to ensure that they have reviewed the program thoroughly and present themselves honestly and in the best light. After the interviews are conducted, students and programs will submit a rank list and hope for the best. Throughout this process faculty and advisors will act as mentors, helping students decide which programs to apply to and how many. Students should listen to these seasoned administrators as they have the best interest of the students in mind and use past experience to guide their decisions. Below are reflections from students currently navigating the residency application process and a reflection from a residency program director.

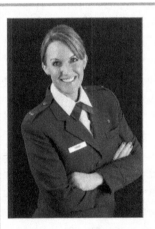

Reflections from a 4th Year Medical Student:
Katherine Tharp, MD, MS
Tarleton State University, MS Counseling
Texas A&M University, BS Journalism
Texas A&M Health Science Center College
* of Medicine, Class of 2015*

My passion for military medicine was ignited before I was ever accepted into medical school. My husband, who is in the Air Force Reserves, was selected for an in-residence Air Force training program in Montgomery, AL, which meant that I was immersed into the life of a military wife. It was the first time I had lived in a military environment and I immediately fell in love with the lifestyle, the airmen, their spouses and children. There was an instant sense of connection and belonging.

I recognized that I was surrounded by an amazing group of people who truly understand sacrifice, in every sense of the word, and are willing to pay a price that so few would voluntarily pay. I have always had a healthy respect for the military, but one-by-one, as I got to know these extraordinary people, this respect morphed into passion and a commitment to do my part. I realized that I wanted to serve those who serve our country.

I started taking my prerequisite courses shortly after we moved to Montgomery. As a non-traditional student with an undergraduate degree in the liberal arts, I had to take all of my science courses. With each course I started, I continued to focus on this population that had become so dear to me. Quite a few years later now with Commissioned Officer Training and Aerospace Medicine training behind me, as well as nearing the finish line for medical school, I am still very much driven to serve in this capacity. To be clear, it has been so nice to have the Air Force pay for my education while also providing a monthly stipend, but I would only encourage joining the military if you have thoroughly researched and are passionate about serving your country.

Most of my medical school experience has been identical to my civilian counterparts. I have had additional education opportunities through the Air Force, but it has not been mandatory. The primary difference between my civilian counterparts and myself became evident fourth year during away rotations and throughout military match. The Air Force requires you do at least one 4-week audition rotation at a residency program where you are interested in matching. Most medical students with a military commitment will actually do two of these rotations. I did 4 weeks at San Antonio Military Medical Center and 4 additional weeks at Wright Patterson Air Force Base. Although there are formal interviews during these rotations, the "interview" is happening everyday. It is a great way to determine goodness of fit between yourself and the program. You are interviewing the program, the other residents, the faculty and staff through your daily interactions, and they in turn, are doing the same thing. That sounds stressful, right? In my situation, I found it to be very relaxed for both rotations. The formal interviews themselves were much like the civilian interviews I attended.

All of the military residency program directors for your chosen specialty will typically meet sometime in November, discuss you, and determine where you match. This means that if you make a really bad impression with one program, all of other program directors will likely know about it. The program directors I interviewed with indicated that they try very hard to place people where they want to be, but at least in the Air Force, those who rank highest on their point system will be given priority.

In my case, there are only two Air Force residencies for psychiatry, so I was able to get to know both programs intimately during my away rotations. However, many students are in specialties that have many more residency programs. In this circumstance, they tend to choose the two they are most interested in placing for their away rotations and then interview with the other programs either in person or via telephone. It is common knowledge that some military residency programs will only chose those students who participated in an away rotation for their slots. Others are more flexible.

One very important distinction between military match and civilian match is the date the results are released. Military match results are released in mid-December whereas civilian match results are typically released mid-March. This is important for a lot of reasons, but I will give you some insight on a few. Most obvious benefit is that you know where you will be living by the end of December. This gives you plenty of time and opportunity for logistical planning and getting to know your new community. It truly is a stress reliever for a lot of individuals.

The military requires that in addition to military match, committed students also apply to the civilian match. I planned my civilian interviews mostly at the end of December and throughout January. It is mandated that you pull out of the civilian match after military match day if you receive a military spot. A substantial sum of money is spent on airfare, car rental, and hotel rooms for each interview, so being able to cancel unnecessary interviews can ultimately save you time, money and anxiety.

I personally ranked "civilian deferred" as my first choice in the military match, followed by the two military programs, in hopes of continuing on at my current institution. Although I am ready to start my career as an Air Force Officer and Physician, I have a husband with some medical issues that would make a move difficult at this time. I was fortunate in that the Air Force had enough psychiatry applicants that they were able to allow me to pursue a civilian residency. This is not always the case, and just like the civilian counterpart, you don't always get your #1 choice.

Although the next 4 years will be spent continuing my formal education in the civilian world, I will start my career as an attending physician in the Air Force immediately post-residency. My commitment to the Air Force is 4 years, but I anticipate loving the work as much as I love the people. My ultimate plan is to continue my career as an Air Force psychiatrist for many years to come. I am so thankful for the opportunity to finish medical school debt free AND be able to spend my professional life giving back to a population of people who, quite frankly, I am honored to know.

continued

Reflections from a 4th Year Medical Student: *(continued)*

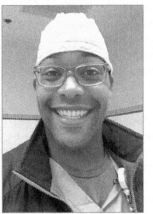

Antoine C. Scott, MD, MS

*Texas A&M Health Science Center College
    of Medicine, Class of 2015*
*University of North Texas Health Science Center,
    MS Medical Science Texas Christian University,
    BA Biology*

It is t-minus 30 days until Match Day, and I am unsure I made the right decision. T-minus 30 and counting until I find out where I will spend the next 5 years of my life training for the long awaited career in medicine. I am not an indecisive person in the least, nor am I one to make emotional or hasty decisions. Yet as anxiety and fear of the unknown sets in, I am forced to answer several questions regarding how exactly I found myself here. And ultimately, have I made the best decision? What was my exposure during medical school that led me to residency selection? What role models/mentors did I encounter along the way? How much of my personality and strengths fit into the specialty I've selected? How far past residency have I attempted to plan out to ensure I have the professional connections to gain a position/fellowship of my choice? What will my career in medicine look like 20 years from now? What follows will be a story of sorts with key questions you should attempt to address when it comes to selecting a residency and, the pursuit of your medical career as a whole.

Exposure: **Has your medical school experience afforded you the breadth of exposure to confidently apply and interview at competitive residency programs?**

Approaching the summit of finishing arguably the most mentally, emotionally, and physically challenging years of my life, of officially becoming Dr. Scott, of seeing the proverbial light at the end of the tunnel, my mind returns back to the day I was accepted into medical school. I remember, unashamedly, flopping onto the hotel bed from exhaustion only to be jolted up with excitement as I read the subject heading from the acceptance email. Full disclosure: that celebration came just off the heels of finishing the day interviewing at another school. It feels so far away from now but, temporally speaking, how proximal it actually was. Why did I choose to train in my particular location? To be completely forthcoming, I chose a place that would offer employment opportunities for my wife, arguably one of the heavier factors in my decision process. I figured, as long as the institution could teach me how to become a doctor, the rest was nonessential. Not knowing that choosing a small college town could impact my exposure to high volumes of severe and complicated patients. Furthermore, even less did I realize that this smaller scale exposure would shape my view of the keystone specialties (Family Practice, Obstetrics/Gynecology, Internal Medicine, Emergency Medicine, Surgery, and Psychiatry). A little background on my exposure to the medical field prior to matriculation; I attended college in Fort Worth, TX, and worked for 2 years scribing for physicians in the ER. Working in hospitals all over the DFW Metroplex, I took for granted the sheer amount of patients I encountered much less the severity of their pathology. That exposure established my baseline and arguably, the exposure during initial years of medical school was subthreshold. However, what a location may lack in patient complexity is more than made up for with the demand of knowledge comprehension on the side of the medical student. Like you all have heard, the courses are hard, study hours are long, and sleep is little. For the didactic months, location mattered much less than step 1 preparation and knowledge mastery. That being said, seeing a complicated patient helps to solidify the clinical application of medical knowledge, the experiential knowledge strengthens neural pathways and supports retention.

Mentor/Role Model: **Have you been able to identify with a current medical doctor who can inform you of the professional landscape? Have you found a physician whom you can emulate and have access to their candid counsel?**

I was born in Texas but raised overseas. My parents were enlistees of the US Army, my childhood spanned across two continents, five countries (including the United States) and five states all within the timespan preceding my 13th birthday. I am the first in my family to attend college, trailblazing as a young black man with a determination to manifest my dream of becoming a doctor. Isolated, ignored, marginalized but never deterred by the challenges and culture shock of this journey to a medical career. I am of the minority in more ways than one. I have never allowed this fact to hold me back or limit the ceiling of my life pursuits. My parents of humble beginnings, to whom I am incredibly grateful, were supportive of my singular dream formed at the early age of seven; they were adamant that I could do anything I put my mind and heart to. What we did not anticipate was that lack of career mentorship or guidance would lead to many uncomfortable and extremely frustrating dead-end experiences. Several times I found the results of my arduous tasks inequitable to my efforts. I painfully had to repeat applications to medical school and MCAT. Each time I learned what my weaknesses were by trying my proverbial hand at the competitive game of medical school matriculation. To grow stronger meant to address my weaknesses head-on and then through almost reverse order, learn what questions I should have asked only after clearing the obstacle. In seeking individuals to emulate, there was paucity of those who shared my background. And, after teasing through the fictional Cliff Huxtables, Christopher Turks, and Eric Foremans, I found no tangible guidance in my sphere of influence for much of my undergraduate and professional school journey. Whether for the disparate numbers of black male physicians in the field or my insufficient search process, I have always been one of few African-American faces encountered since attending college on academic scholarship. But I digress, medical school was no different, often times I felt all the twinges of doubt from the sheer challenge of my studies further complicated by a strong sense of isolation and loneliness. Whether it was social discrepancy with my presence, my eagerness to connect or simply being misunderstood, I established few lasting friendships in medical school. To combat this and hopefully garner strong colleagues, I involved myself with the governance of my student class body and joined the electorate leadership. Attending AAMC conferences exposed me to the pedagogy of medical education. It also allowed me to meet other minority medical students around the nation offering a stronger network of support. Still I yearned for a mentor, no longer requiring them to look like me, just desiring them see the eager student I was and take me under their wing; introduce me to the apprenticeship of medicine. Focusing so hard on matriculating to medical school and excelling in my coursework, I never really had the time to slow down and ask, "What type of doctor do I want to be?" I was the pluripotent stem cell waiting for the surge of electricity spurring my differentiation down a fated lineage. I came to medical school open to becoming any type of physician, ready to master the coursework, make study group partners, sleep little, and let serendipity and inspiration strike me where they may. I did not know the process of selecting a specialty was so fluid, that there was no formula (and if there was, I had no idea where to find it). So being nondiscriminatory toward all specialties, I looked to interest groups partially for free food but also hoping to be met with a distinct sense of affirmation. I joined several groups and remain engaged in the seeking process, but how many interest groups can you be in before you just seem disinterested in making a decision? Third year clinicals came and went, I began to strike off several specialties. But still, factoring in my summer research experiences, several specialties remained in my top five. In the end, it took the encouragement and candid counsel of a particular vascular surgeon and faculty member to affirm my choice to become a surgeon. I could handle the rigor, I am an early morning person by nurture, and I enjoyed the challenge of applying anatomy and physiology with surgical technique. The rest was nonessential, so I thought.

continued

Reflections from a 4th Year Medical Student: *(continued)*

Personality/Strengths Fit: **How competitive are your scores for this specialty? Is this specialty aligned with your natural strengths and abilities? Are you pursuing a specialty for reasons intrinsic or extrinsic to your motivations? What experience or individual is driving you to pursue this specialty? Does your personality mesh with the ones within that specialty field?**

Reluctantly, I honed my lone-wolf experience and found myself gravitating to the challenges of Surgery. Encountering the operating room brought back fond memories of my favorite course, gross anatomy. I found the toughest yet fun personalities along with the most decisive minds. And, I much preferred the operating room setting to any other medical setting previously experienced. The patient interactions were unlike any other. Frankly, I mostly enjoyed the teamwork and interacting with the personalities on both sides of the sterile field. It was there that I saw a way to gain the respect and admiration of my colleagues.

Trajectory Beyond Residency/Connections: **How will this residency assist you in tailor-making your career in medicine? What are your hobbies/interests outside of medicine and, how will this residency/specialty allow you to pursue them in the future? What priorities influence your decision for selecting this residency?**

I had never thought further than my residency start date until I found myself in a metropolitan city with diverse medical staff and complex patients with advanced pathology. Each of the previously ignored specialties seemed ratcheted up several notches close to the point of being interesting. I appreciated the many nuances of OB/GYN, the complex treatments of Psychiatry, the exciting rounds of Internal Medicine, and the pharmacological orchestration of Anesthesia. I was experiencing a whole new side to every specialty. Through my fourth-year electives in Houston, I encountered African-American physicians excited about their status in the workplace and medical career, eager to pass on their wisdom and life experiences. It was so enriching. For the first time I, internally, was able to exhale deeply and enjoy the process of medical school. I finally felt accepted. The hours were much tougher but my satisfaction so much greater. Now with my marriage being in its fourth year, my wife and I felt ready to expand our family and I felt able to consider the long-term ramifications of my medical career choices. Even as I write this, things are less in limbo yet still to be determined, Match Day cometh and I am excited for the future.

There will come a time when your vocation becomes a job, a job you strived your entire life to fulfill, nonetheless, a job. Whatever challenges and triumphs you face on your march toward residency, I hope you experience something that makes you think beyond residency years down the road when your calling becomes less of your identity, when your life is enriched by your own familial investments. What led me down this road? I cannot mark each milestone or dead-end experience, but what I can say is that my adventure so far has taught me several things along the way. These are not answers to the great algorithm of residency selection, simply my checklist of questions; questions that empower you to make the best decision possible with the amount of information available to you.

1. Has your medical school experience afforded you the breadth of exposure to confidently apply and interview at competitive residency programs?
2. Have you been able to identify with a current medical doctor who can inform you of the professional landscape?
3. Have you found a physician whom you can emulate and have access to their candid counsel?
4. How competitive are your scores for this specialty?
5. Is this specialty aligned with your natural strengths and abilities?

6. Are you pursuing a specialty reasons intrinsic or extrinsic to your motivations?
7. What experience or individual is driving you to pursue this specialty?
8. Does your personality mesh with the ones within that specialty field?
9. How will this residency assist you in tailor-making your career in medicine?
10. What are your hobbies/interests outside of medicine and, how will this residency/specialty allow you to pursue to them in the future?
11. What priorities influence your decision for selecting this residency?

Final Pointers

The Application—If money and time availability permit, apply to a broad range of programs to increase your probabilities of matching into your specialty. Apply for away rotations in locations you would want to match into.

Interviewing—The lionshare of this information will come from a good understanding of who you are as a potential candidate, knowing what you contribute to the composition of the intern class, strong study of your CV, and having concrete expectations for the program of interest. Knowing how to sell your strengths comes from articulating your professional assets and extracurricular hobbies. Be professional and engaged.

The Match—Simply the by-product of putting the best version of you on display and keeping record of places you best fit.

© Kendall Hunt Publishing Company

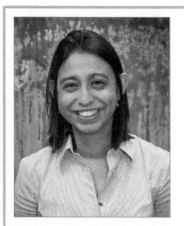

Mo Som, DO, MS

Clinical Assistant Professor of Internal Medicine

Internal Medicine Residency Program Director, Oklahoma State University, Center for Health Sciences

Medical School, University of North Texas Health Science Center, Texas College of Osteopathic Medicine

College, University of Arizona

As an Internal Medicine Program Director, the most desirable candidates are the ones that we feel are the most trainable. By the end of 3 years, we have to feel comfortable knowing that our graduates are prepared for whatever walks through the door; whether it be in the ICU, on the wards, in Fellowship, or in the outpatient clinic. While board scores and GPA are important to us as initial screening tools, they will only take them so far in their career and we recognize it is what they do with these numbers that count. We look for candidates that may be able to recite page 1920 of Harrisons but can also sit at the bedside and know that page 1920 doesn't matter to the patient or their family.

Audition rotations serve as the foundation for our vetting process. We look to see how they interact with their patients, peers, residents, and faculty. We gauge their progress through the month to see how quickly they assimilate themselves into a busy

continued

(continued)

service. During this month we try to determine if the candidate can be trained in the art of medicine and not just plug patients into an algorithm.

And finally the Interview; this serves as the last step in our selection process. Core faculty and chief residents review the candidate's entire application from their performance in medical school to their letters of recommendation and personal statement while visiting with them in a setting that is outside of clinical rounds. This last piece helps us tie it all together and gives us a glimpse of the person underneath the white coat.

© Kendall Hunt Publishing Company

Chapter 10
Graduate Medical Education (Residency and Fellowship)

Medical Residency Training

Medical students spend four years (or more depending on additional education) attaining knowledge and trying to reach graduation. Their first year of medical school is full of idealism and wonder as well as stress and overwhelming amounts of information. The introduction to medical education can be equated to drinking from a fire

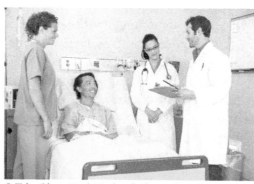

© Tyler Olson, 2014. Used under license from Shutterstock, Inc.

hydrant. Then, students enter second year and they are a bit more jaded, but recognize that although their workload has increased they can handle it. At the beginning of their third year, students usually gain a renewed sense of purpose because they are finally doing what they came to medical school to do, participating in the clinical setting and taking care of patients. This is a stressful yet exciting year because students are solidifying their career choices. However, this year often comes with a different form of jade, which is often a reflection of negativity from clinicians. The negativity observed is often in a form of both implicit and explicit biases that students witness. Finally, fourth year begins and students have a mixed sense of excitement and anxiety. Excitement because fourth year is the first time that students experience some flexibility in medical school, and they are doing exactly what they want to do, participating in a medical specialty that excites them. Overall, this year gives students time to self reflect and relax. However, this light at the end of the tunnel is quickly met with the reality of the next step in their journey of medical education: Residency.

Residency is the student's first venture as a physician. Residency time frames vary depending on specialty and residency requirements. Some specialties take longer to master than others and some programs have begun to require an extra year for research. Resident physicians receive progressive responsibility until they are able to be fully responsible for patient care. Also of note is that the USMLE or COMLEX Step 3 is taken during residency (at the end of internship year).

Now that the word **internship** is out there, it is important to clarify that residency includes an internship year. This internship year can be part of the residency program or it can be separate from the program. When the internship is separate, it is often called a preliminary or transitional year.

Specialties that sometimes require a preliminary year (separate internship year) are: anesthesia, radiology, dermatology, and ophthalmology.

The last type of residency spot is a **categorical** spot. Categorical is most often utilized in the primary care training. The student will match into one spot and stay in that spot until graduating from residency.

Specialty Choice

Many students struggle with specialty choice and one of the first things a student should ask themselves is do they want to be procedure or not procedure oriented. The reason to use procedure rather than surgical is because many students assume working with their hands has to be surgical, but instead can be procedural. Working with their hands can include subspecialties like cardiology, pulmonary/critical care, interventional radiology, and gastroenterology are also hands-on specialties. It is also important to factor in the desire for patient interaction. There are a few specialties that do not require much patient interaction and these are perfect for the student who enjoys the field of medicine, but does not necessarily enjoy traditional clinical medicine. Pathology and radiology are most common for this student.

Procedure/Surgical	Non-Procedure/ Clinical	Mixed
Colon and Rectal Surgery	Medical Genetics	Obstetrics and Gynecology
Emergency Medicine	Pathology	Dermatology
General Surgery	Preventative Medicine	Ophthalmology
Neurology	Radiation Oncology	Internal Medicine (Inpatient Medicine)
Orthopaedic Surgery	Family Medicine	
Thoracic Surgery	Radiology	
Anesthesiology	Psychiatry	
Otolaryngology (ENT)	Pediatrics	
Plastic Surgery	Radiology	
Urology		

(Not all specialties and subspecialties are listed.)

Life as a Resident

Life as a resident is similar to the metamorphosis that occurs throughout medical school. The resident starts out as the low man/woman on the totem poll the July after they graduate from medical school. Many residents have much anxiety about practicing as a doctor "on their own" and what they do not realize is that they are not on their own. Instead they are under many layers of supervision; their supervision consists of an upper level resident, sometimes a fellow, and then an attending physician. In addition to all of these physicians, experienced nurses and physician assistants often serve as a wealth of knowledge for the intern. It is often stated that good nurses keep young doctors from killing patients. Obviously, a comment said in jest, but it illustrates the value of allied health care professionals. Once a student progresses to their second year of residency, they feel a little more confident in their skills and are given a bit more responsibility. This process is three to five years depending on the type of residency program chosen. With each year comes more training and more autonomy.

"Suck it up, work hard and it will be over; do it all and don't hold back. There is something to learn in everything." This is a quote from a physician about internship year. He also said, "I wouldn't wish internship year on anybody."

Primary care training (internal medicine, family medicine, pediatrics) normally takes three years, while surgical specialities often take longer—five or more years. Keep in mind that many people go on to do fellowships after residency to further specialize, and this takes extra time, requires another test (board certification), as well as additional years of trainee salary.

Although the salary is minimal compared to the hours worked, residents and fellows do receive a small raise each year and some seniority. Residents start out making on average mid–high $30s to low $40s and receive a 1 to 3 thousand dollar raise each year. The amounts depend on the programs. As the resident's responsibility increases, their organization and confidence increases as well, so the years seem to get better. With this new confidence, he/she will notice that the program becomes less physically demanding, but progressively more mentally demanding. However, the renewed confidence that the resident feels in their role allows them to adapt well to the additional responsibility.

First Year

First year residents often have a set of required rotations—some are within their chosen specialty and others are outside. For instance, an internal medicine resident, will most likely rotate in an inpatient (hospital) setting, outpatient (clinic) setting, in the intensive care unit, and often within other specialties like emergency medicine, and subspecialties like gastroenterology and nephrology. This is set up to ensure well-rounded training and give the intern a robust amount of knowledge to draw from in their future training. Interns are expected to absorb vast amounts of information and to read as much as possible. Ideally, reading every night about something seen within the day.

An intern is essentially an information gatherer; still not quite getting the big picture, but doing their best to learn as much as possible.

Second Year +

By the time second year starts, residents are starting to see the bigger picture, which is good because the expectations are a bit more involved. During second year, a resident will be expected to take on a leadership role. The resident may be expected to lead a team with an intern and other health care professionals. Part of leading this team is management of the team and management of the patient. The resident must now go beyond data gathering and start to create a plan for patient management. If the resident is at a teaching institution, they will also be expected to do some teaching for those on the team. Responsibility will only increase as the training program goes on. Some programs will expect their residents to take on research and teaching roles on a more consistent basis.

Final year

In the final year of residency, the physician is feeling confident and successfully doing everything that was expected in year two and three, etc., but something new has been added to that list: deciding on a future. There are several paths that the physician can take: go into private practice, choose more training and complete a fellowship, participate in academic medicine, or complete a chief year that often helps propel a career in administration. Because the future is imminent, residents look for autonomy and opportunities to ensure they are ready for their next step.

If a resident chooses to go out into practice, they have several decisions to make about what type of medicine they are interested in—clinic or hospital medicine or both. Would they like to focus on something within their practice? Will they be joining a group, working for a hospital, or . . .? Will they choose to be in academics? These are all questions that the resident will have to answer as they choose their next step.

Just as there are many questions to be asked when choosing the right practice, the same is true when choosing a fellowship. Many trainees know that they want to subspecialize by the second year of residency. If they choose this path, then they will be required to participate in the match process again. With this process comes the interviews and researching programs.

Finally, there is a less common option of doing a chief year. This is a year of serving as a junior faculty in administration. It is often used to make an application more appealing or competitive for fellowships. It can also be seen as a good move to jump-start a career in administration. The use of a chief year is not universal, however. Some surgical specialties have chief residents in the last year of their residency rather than it being an extra year. Some are elected while others are chief by virtue of being in their last year of residency. It will be important to review what each program means by chief year to ensure understanding of their definition.

Additional Requirements

Some additional requirements for residency may be research, participation in lunch educational sessions, morning meetings, journal clubs, and creating presentations.

- **Research Requirement** – Could range from presenting a poster at an in-house research day to a peer-reviewed publication.
- **Lunch Education Sessions** – Some programs may have an attendance requirement and mandate a percentage of attendance. Due to work hour restrictions, some programs have started using the lunch hour to educate their residents with lunch lectures. Faculty within the department present or external speakers present. Upper-level residents are often asked to participate in presenting as well.
- **Journal Club** – This is the act of reviewing current articles also known as evidence. It is normally done in groups over a meal. Many programs have a journal club and some require attendance and/or a presentation at journal club. Journal club is part of the application of Evidence Based Medicine. As programs move to be evidence based, journal club becomes more and more popular. The format of journal club differs from group to group, but the major purpose is to review new articles and critique the article for future practice. Questions may be asked such as "Does the article have clinically significant findings that should change the way we practice?" The best way to get everyone invested is to provide food and to have the participants take part in choosing what they read.[1]
- **Presentations** – Some programs require that residents give noon lectures. This could be on a topic or over a case that he/she has seen.

Typical Day for an Internal Medicine Intern

For an intern, a typical day on the inpatient service would start with looking up every patient and their labs to ensure readiness to present the patient to the team and attendings during rounds. Rounds is a term that is used to describe what the team does first when arriving in the morning. The team gathers and discusses each patient briefly before they visit that patient and make a further assessment. Rounds take most of the morning and can even go beyond that time frame. It depends upon the team leader, patient acuity, and patient load. Following rounds, lunch lectures are often required. This is when staff or residents present new information or evidence for practice. Many programs require the residents to conduct research and literature reviews for these presentations. Following lunch, residents spend time discharging patients, admitting patients, and following up on orders.

---

[1] EBM Notebook . . . . . . What makes evidence-based journal clubs succeed? www.evidence -basedmedicine.com http://ebm.bmj.com/content/9/2/36.full.pdf+html

Morning meetings and five o'clock meetings can also add to a long day. Many programs have morning meetings because it is the best time to catch everyone. Some surgical programs meet before starting their day, which might be earlier than other specialties.

Example Day as an Intern:
• 6:00 a.m. – arrive at the hospital and review patients for rounds • 8:00 a.m. – start rounding with the team • 12:00 p.m. – lunch meeting/lecture • 1:00 p.m. – work on discharge, admits, and follow-ups • 6:00ish p.m. – leave OR . . . go to journal club

As though this schedule is not busy enough, a resident is also expected to find time to conduct research. As stated above, some programs require presentations; others require posters for their in-house research day, and some go as far as to require conference submissions and publications. Research as a requirement is becoming more and more of a norm. Many programs are very open about their requirement, which can be found on their website or the FREIDA site.

The best way to accomplish this research requirement is to find a mentor within the program and be a part of their research. Some programs may even assign a research mentor. If one is not assigned, it is important for a resident to find one as they will educate and help the resident through the institutional processes (both formal and informal). This process can be used as a medical student as well. Many medical students have published during medical school because they were able to find an excellent mentor who ensured publication. Finally, participation in research can also help one be more marketable or desirable for fellowship programs.

Call and Tests

Much of a resident's call will be in-house. This is where the original term of "house officer" was derived. Long ago residents actually lived at the hospital. Now, there are rules against overworking residents (ACGME work hours). Despite these new rules, sleep continues to elude the resident while on call because the pager seems to go off just as he/she is drifting to sleep. The sleep that they do get is not sound as the concern of the pager going off at any second lingers in the mind. As the resident becomes more comfortable and confident, sleep becomes easier.

There are several tests that are taken during residency. Interns take the USMLE Step 3 or COMLEX; there is an in-service exam that most residency programs give, jurisprudence (JP) exam, and board exam that provides board certification. Step 3 is the final Step exam (remember USMLE Step 1, Step 2 CK and CS, or COMLEX Level 1 and Level 2 CE & PE from Chapter 5) and is taken during the intern year. The in-service exam is not universal, but if the program chooses to use it, then it may be given as often as annually. The JP exam is one that many people disregard and cram for, but it is a requirement for board certification within the state of Texas. It does not require a huge amount of study, but it must be passed. The board examination will vary depending on specialty. For example, internal medicine boards are written (computer-based), while other specialties such as radiol-

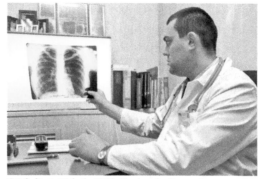

© Vladimir Melnik, 2014. Used under license from Shutterstock, Inc.

ogy and orthopedics require oral boards as well as written. Some even require that you collect your own patients for review. If a sub-specialty is chosen, then the resident will have additional board examinations. Just as step examinations cost money, so do the board examinations.

Life as a resident involves sacrifice. Residents miss out on time and holidays with friends and family. Often family and friends cannot begin to understand the sacrifices their loved-one makes to be a physician. This is why physicians often stick together within their friend circle. Not because they are too arrogant to be around others, but instead because they do not have to worry about the judgment and assumptions of others. In these circles, they are able to lament about patient issues without feeling bad, they are also able to vent without someone saying, "It must be nice." or something frustrating.

With these things in mind, if a simple thank you from a patient or patient's family along with the intrinsic motivation to help people is enough to keep a resident motivated, then he/she will make it and be happy they did. Most physicians do not go into medicine for the money, but instead because they felt like it was their calling. Remaining passionate about work through all of these challenges may mean the right choice was made.

Residents who have chosen a sub-specialty to follow residency training will go through the application process once again. Those who want to pursue a fellowship complete the application process in their last year of residency. This process is the same match process that was conducted for residency.

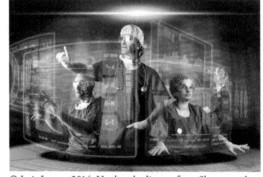

© Luis Louro, 2014. Used under license from Shutterstock, Inc.

Unfortunately for the resident, they become low man on the totem pole all over again. The anxiety of the unknown is back and the senior resident becomes a first-year fellow. As a first-year fellow, metamorphosis begins again. The difference this time is that the physician most likely has completed boards and has done this once before, so he/she is more confident in their ability to learn and grow in the process.

Fellowship, like residency, varies in length. There are fellowships that last one, two, or three years. There are also fellowships that can be tacked on to multiple specialties. For example, sports medicine can be added to a family medicine or an orthopaedics residency. One would be more focused on the surgical aspect than the other. Another fellowship that can follow multiple residencies is critical care. All of the following can be the first step prior to a critical care fellowship: Emergency Medicine + Critical Care, Internal Medicine + Critical Care, Anesthesia + Critical Care, Surgery + Critical Care . . . There are a number of ways to accomplish ultimate goals. Oncology is another fellowship that can be done following different residencies: Surgery + Oncology, Internal Medicine + Oncology . . .

This is important to remember when choosing a path. For example, if the student knows they want to do critical care and that they prefer being in the operating room (OR) as opposed to the clinic, then they will most likely want to choose a residency that is primarily in the OR.

Something else to keep in mind is that there are also apprentice opportunities that have not yet become accredited fellowships. These are usually an additional year of training beyond the chosen specialty.

Because there are so many options out there and a limited amount of time in medical school to preview all options, it is important that a student do his/her research and go beyond shadowing one or two doctors. If this is done and a student truly understands what their chosen profession is about, then it is evident within the interview. This is true within any interview (for medical school, for residency, and for fellowship). When the interviewee is knowledgeable and well-versed about their chosen profession, it is impressive and refreshing.

Fellowships

As mentioned before, keep in mind that not all fellowship programs have registered with the NRMP.

NRMP Registered Programs:
Abdominal Transplant Surgery, Adolescent Medicine, Allergy/
    Immunology,
Pediatric Anesthesiology, Pain Medicine, Colon & Rectal Surgery,
    Hand Surgery,
Female Pelvic Medicine and Reconstructive Surgery, Geriatric Medicine,
Laryngology, Medical Genetics, Cardiovascular Disease, Endocrinology,
Gastroenterology, Hematology/Oncology, Infectious Disease,
    Interventional
Pulmonology, Nephrology, Oncology, Pulmonary, Pulmonary and
    Critical Care,
Rheumatology, Medical Toxicology, Neonatal-Perinatal Medicine,
    Gynecologic
Oncology, Maternal-Fetal Medicine, Minimally Invasive Gynecologic
    Surgery,
Pediatric and Adolescent Gynecology, Reproductive Endocrinology,
    Pediatric

Hematology/Oncology, Pediatric Rehabilitation Medicine,
Developmental-Behavioral Pediatrics, Pediatric Critical Care
Medicine, Pediatric Emergency
Medicine, Pediatric Nephrology, Pediatric Rheumatology, Pediatric
Cardiology,
Pediatric Endocrinology, Pediatric Gastroenterology, Pediatric Infectious
Diseases,
Pediatric Pulmonology, Pediatric Surgery, Primary Care Sports
Medicine, Child and
Adolescent Psychiatry, Psychosomatic Medicine, Interventional
Radiology,
Neuroradiology, Sleep Medicine, Surgical Critical Care, Thoracic
Surgery, Vascular Surgery

Two fellowships that come to mind that aren't listed are within Orthopaedics. Trauma and sports medicine are common fellowships for residents that go into Orthopaedics and yet they are not part of the NRMP, so it is conceivable that what you want is out there and not listed with this match system. This again highlights the importance of seeking out a mentor in the field. This person can expose you to things that you did not even know existed.

JAMA PATIENT PAGE   The Journal of the American Medical Association

MEDICAL EDUCATION

Medical Specialties

Future physicians go to **medical school** after they complete college. Medical students learn about many different areas of medicine, including those designated as specialties. At the end of medical school, doctors choose the specialty in which they will have more education and eventually practice. Education in each specialty takes 3 to 7 years of a residency after medical school. Some medical specialties have **subspecialties** that require even more education and training. Since medical knowledge is so complex and advanced, most doctors limit their practices to their area of specialization. The September 7, 2011, issue of *JAMA* is a theme issue on medical education. This Patient Page is based on one previously published in the September 5, 2007, issue of *JAMA*.

PRIMARY CARE SPECIALTIES
- Family medicine (primary care of adults and children)
- Internal medicine (primary care of adults)
- Pediatrics (primary care of children)

Doctors who practice in the primary care specialties focus on general care of the patient. They often coordinate the specialized care that a patient may receive from different medical specialists. Primary care physicians usually provide continuing care for patients over a long time. They are also concerned with preventing diseases and medical problems.

OTHER SPECIALTIES

- Allergy and immunology
- Anesthesiology (pain control and other care during surgery)
- Colon and rectal surgery
- Dermatology
- Emergency medicine
- Medical genetics
- Neurology (diseases of the nervous system)
- Neurosurgery (surgery of the brain and nervous system)
- Nuclear medicine (use of nuclear materials in diagnosis and treatment)
- Obstetrics and gynecology (female reproductive system including prenatal and birth care)

- Ophthalmology (eye diseases)
- Orthopedic surgery (bones and joints)
- Otolaryngology (ear, nose, and throat)
- Pathology (diagnosis of tissues and body fluids)
- Physical medicine and rehabilitation
- Plastic surgery (reconstructive and cosmetic surgery)
- Preventive medicine
- Psychiatry
- Radiology (diagnosis using images; radiation therapy)
- Surgery
- Thoracic surgery (chest and heart surgery)
- Urology (kidneys and urinary system)

SUBSPECIALTIES

Examples of subspecialties of internal medicine and pediatrics include **cardiology** (heart disease), **nephrology** (kidney diseases), and **rheumatology** (arthritis and connective tissue diseases). Examples of surgical subspecialties include **hand surgery** and **vascular** (blood vessel) **surgery**.

Information on specialties can be obtained from the **American Board of Medical Specialties**, an organization that regulates the development of specialties in medicine. This organization upholds the standards that allow doctors to become **board certified**. When a doctor meets all the requirements of a medical specialty board (a required level of education, experience, and specialized testing of knowledge and skill), she or he is called a diplomate of that specialty board. The doctor is then allowed to state that she or he is board certified in that medical specialty. A doctor's board certification can be verified through the American Board of Medical Specialties.

FOR MORE INFORMATION
- American Board of Medical Specialties www.abms.org
- Council of Medical Specialty Societies www.cmss.org

INFORM YOURSELF

To find this and previous JAMA Patient Pages, go to the Patient Page link on *JAMA*'s Web site at www.jama.com. Many are available in English and Spanish.

Sources: American Board of Medical Specialties, American Medical Association, Council of Medical Specialty Societies

Janet M. Torpy, MD, Writer

Robert M. Golub, MD, Editor

From, *The Journal of the American Medical Association*, Volume 298, Number 9 (September 5, 2007). Reprinted by permission.

Reflections from a Resident

By Marcelo D. Ribeiro, MD
Resident, Scott & White Radiology,
Temple, TX, 2012–2017
Texas A&M Health Science Center College of
Medicine, Class of 2012
University of Texas at Arlington,
Bachelor of Science in Nursing, 2004
Radiology Resident, Scott & White Health Care
System

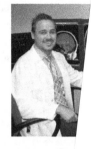

A combination of factors led me to choose radiology as my career. First a
importantly, I had to choose a field that I enjoy and could truly picture
in for the rest of my life. Other factors such as the personality of individuals
been in the field for 5, 10, 20+ years matching up with mine was also paramount because
I wanted to go into a field where I would "fit in." Individual talents and shortcomings are
also very important to consider. For me, I'm a visual learner. I like a rapid and repetitive
flow to my work and enjoy working with my hands, which is why radiology is a good fit
and why I feel that fellowship training in interventional radiology will be a perfect fit.

I originally came into medical school wanting to be a surgeon. In fact, I had wanted
to be a pediatric cardiothoracic surgeon since I was in elementary school because I have a
passion for congenital heart defects. So, initially, I had my "blinders" on and was very
close-minded to other fields. When I rotated through surgery during my third year of
medical school, I slowly came to an unexpected realization—I liked surgery, but I didn't
LOVE it. To me, it was very important to come out doing something I LOVED if I was
going to spend the first three decades of my life pursuing a specific goal.

So, after surgery rotation, I lost the "blinders" and began looking for my new
passion. When I had exposure to radiology and more specifically to interventional
radiology, I had my "Aha, THIS is what I'm supposed to be doing for the rest of my
life" moment. And the more exposure I had and the more I researched the field, the
more confident I became in my decision.

There are several key differences between medical school and residency. If you've
ever had a job with a boss that expected you to show up on time and do your work and
then go home, you're ahead of the curve! The hierarchy of residency is something that I
feel is unique to medicine and some business fields. In residency, you start out as an
intern (a.k.a. the "bottom of the totem pole"), and then move on to be a resident, then
an upper-level resident, then a fellow (if you undergo additional specialty training after
your initial residency), and finally become the attending physician. In most residencies,
interns are expected to initially voice questions and/or concerns to the resident that is
"above" them, then that upper-level resident can ask his/her fellow the question if they
don't know the answer, and finally the fellow can ask the attending if they require
clarification. This may seem highly inefficient, but this actually serves a very practical
purpose in medicine. You see, it allows the person that most recently learned the
answer to your question to answer it, thus reinforcing his/her learning. This is not to
say that you aren't allowed to look your attending in the eyes and ask a question if
you're an intern, just don't be surprised if your attending asks another resident to
answer your question before they expand on it and give you a little bedside teaching
session full of pearls of wisdom.

Resident life is hectic, but it's good. It's like medical school in the regard that
you're still learning, reading, and taking care of patients. But it's not like medical
school in the fact that you aren't taking tests all the time, studying into the wee hours
of the morning, and lastly . . . drumroll please . . . you get a PAYCHECK!! And
although its not a large paycheck, it does allow you to live in a nice apartment or house,
drive a reliable car, and take your significant other on a date on Saturday nights.

In residency, I enjoy meeting new people, whether it is the patients, their family
members, other residents, attendings, and other members of the health care team such

(continued)

as nurses and respiratory therapists. Developing a good rapport with others by having a good attitude towards all team members goes a long way and makes the long hours and intellectual demands enjoyable. I also enjoy seeing patients take a turn for the better, and the gratitude they have towards you when you help them get to a better state of health is truly priceless and makes all the hard work very worth it.

The biggest challenge for me has been the steep learning curve that is seen in residency. No matter how hard you study or how well you do in medical school, residency is a different environment where you must now learn all of the different aspects specific to your specialty. Initially, you may feel like you don't know anything and are just trying to play catch-up. But once you have a few months under your belt, things become easier and you'll impress yourself with how much you are picking up "on the fly."

My last little tidbit of advice about medical school, residency, etc., is if you have a dream, just go for it! Time is going to pass by whether you're pursuing your dreams or not. And whether you are successful in your pursuits or not, one day you'll look back and have succeeded, be content that you tried, or be kicking yourself for not trying. One of my favorite quotes that I heard long ago is: "If you never give up, you will ultimately not fail." I think that's a powerful motto to live your life by, no matter what your dream.

Reflections from Fellows

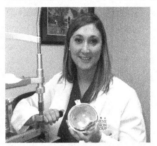

By Michele Riggins, MD
Neuro-Ophthalmologist, Grene Vision Group,
*   Wichita, KS, 2012 –present*
Dean McGee Eye Institute, Neuro-Ophthalmology
*   Fellowship, Oklahoma City, OK, 2011–2012*
Scott and White Hospital Ophthalmology Residency,
*   Temple, TX, 2008–2011*
Scott and White Hospital Internal Medicine Preliminary
*   Year, Temple, TX, 2007–2008*
Texas A&M Health Science Center College of Medicine, Class of 2007 Texas A&M
University, BS in Biomedical Science, 2002

Each decision along my medical career was a difficult one, not because I am a naturally indecisive person, but because of the pressure to choose wisely. Deciding to do a fellowship encouraged me to broadly brainstorm over three categories: time, money, and job satisfaction.

Much time is needed to become a practicing doctor, even before a fellowship is tacked on at the end. I know quite a few people that have even done more than one fellowship. While in residency, I could see that illusive light at the end of the tunnel, so, mentally, even thinking about extending that training time can be very taxing. More time needs to be spent researching which type of fellowship is best (such as deciding between a retina fellowship and a surgical neuro-ophthalmology fellowship, which was in my case). Much time is needed to then research where to do the fellowship and to make connections at those places. Personal connections are vital, because they help to give an idea about the possible personalities and settings at a particular location, and whether that matches up with the fellow. Time is needed to actually interview at these places, and then, of course, the time required to complete the fellowship needs considered. I could handle one more year, as my fellowship was just that short. Some fellowships are at least three years and can seem to double the training time spent after medical school. If the time seems to be a deterrent, both money and job satisfaction also need to be considered, as a small sacrifice now might be best.

Let us all be honest. Before getting into medical school, money is contemplated in some fashion. Money pays the bills and then some. For the most part, a fellowship-trained physician could be salaried more money than their comprehensive counterparts.

Reflections from Fellows *(continued)*

This needs to be weighed against the time it takes to arrive there. Again, my fellowship in neuro-ophthalmology was a year, and I could handle living on a fellow's salary for that long. I was able to start to pay back the medical school loans while in fellowship, but that may prove difficult when there are more mouths to feed; hence, the time spent while in fellowship can be very costly for a family, especially the longer fellowships. The fellowship and time spent completing it is not the only money needing to be considered. Some fellowships will not be offered at the place of residency, meaning a move is necessary. Moving can be pricey, as is interviewing for the extra training can be costly with flights and hotel. I limited my interviews to three to keep the cost down, but an ultra-competitive fellowship may require more places to ensure that one is accepted, making the price tag high. For me, the money spent getting into a fellowship, the money earned while in fellowship, and the salary garnered after being a fellowship-trained doctor was completely worth it, and this added to my job satisfaction.

Money is definitely a motivating factor, but if a doctor is miserable every morning, dreading to go to work, then some might argue that money may not be worth it. Job satisfaction was my most important factor that I considered. I am realistic and know that there will always be a bad day in the business, but I wanted to wake up and want to come to work a majority of days. I had to decide if I was satisfied being the doctor that referred patients to a specialist, or if I wanted to be that specialist. I wanted that daily challenge, the person that my colleagues would inquire for my professional expert opinion. I also was not sure if I wanted to be in a teaching position or private practice, and being fellowship-trained, I can do both at some point in my career. Looking back, any question that arose prior to deciding to go for a fellowship could be categorized in the time, money, or job satisfaction zones. Keeping fewer categories and somewhat simplifying the decision-making process definitely gave me a clear idea of what my next step should be, because, as stated above, I was not the most decisive person.

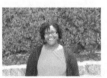

By Nanette Allison, DO, MS
Attending Physician at MHMR of Tarrant County, 2013–present
University of Texas Southwestern Medical Center Child/
*   Adolescent Psychiatry, 2011–2013*
John Peter Smith Hospital Psychiatry Residency, 2007–2011
University of North Texas Health Science Center, Texas College of Osteopathic
*   Medicine, 2007*
Baylor University, BA in Biology, 2002

Deciding to complete a fellowship program was a big decision for me. I was in my last year of a rigorous psychiatry residency, and was looking forward to graduating and beginning my career as an attending physician. I was advised by many about the money I would lose by extending my training and committing to a two-year fellowship program (i.e., the salary of an attending is about three times that of a resident), but I knew in my heart of hearts that I wanted to be a child and adolescent psychiatrist. I sat down and created a list of pros and cons. Pros: I would be able to work with children. I would also be more marketable, because I would be a double-boarded psychiatrist (general and child/adolescent). There was also the potential for a higher starting salary since this sub-specialty was in high demand. The major cons included two more years of a trainee's salary, two more years of intense and demanding night/weekend call, and my student loans would continue to accrue interest since they would stay in deferment and/or forbearance.

Now that I have completed my fellowship, there is no doubt in my mind that I made the right choice. Even though there were many long days, I enjoyed the education I received. Upon graduation, I was able to secure a position as an outpatient child psychiatrist and had many offers to choose from. I am enjoying my new position as an attending psychiatrist and continue to know that I made the right choice by completing a fellowship.

Go to the following website: http://www.med-ed.virginia.edu/specialties/.
Take the Medical Specialty Aptitude Test.

Which specialty was the result?

What are your thoughts on this specialty? Do you think it is a good reflection
of you?

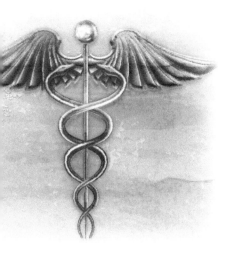

Chapter 11
The Practice of Medicine

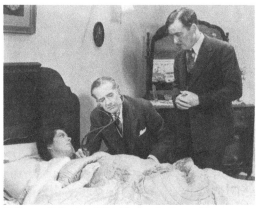

© Everett Collection, 2014. Used under license from Shutterstock, Inc.

Gone are the days of house calls, doctors traveling in covered wagons to see their patients, and receiving a chicken or eggs as payment for their services. The things that have not changed are the hours and dedication that being a physician requires. These requirements vary between specialties, but as mentioned in a previous chapter the training is intense no matter the chosen specialty.

Once a physician has chosen their specialty, he/she is then tasked with finding the right type of practice. The practice of medicine is extraordinarily diverse. A physician can choose to work in several settings. Some options include academic centers like the Mayo Clinic in Rochester, MN, a hospital group, which can be any hospital that does not affiliate with an educational institution, a large clinic, a small office, or any combination of the aforementioned.

The specialty of choice will dictate the blueprint of future medical practice. Primary care specialties are often in clinical practices with a smaller amount of hospital work, while surgical specialties will require access to a hospital. However, this is not always the case, especially if a primary care physician decides to become a hospitalist, someone who chooses to work in the hospital as an inpatient doctor, or if he/she decides to complete a fellowship requiring more hospital work. Many specialties, particularly within Internal Medicine, involve minimally invasive procedures typically done in an outpatient setting. These procedures require some sort of surgical suite (i.e., cardiac catheterization lab, endoscopy suite, or bronchoscopy suite).

Hospital versus clinical work is not the only dichotomy within practice. Two other dichotomies are academic versus non-academic and private versus not-private practice. These three dichotomies make the practice of medicine extraordinarily diverse because one choice does not preclude another. It is possible to be a hospitalist in private practice who participates in academic medicine. Even if a physician chooses a non-academic institution, it is still possible to seek an opportunity to participate in medical education within the community.

Hospital vs. Clinic

Most specialties have a mixture of clinic and hospital responsibilities. For example, a surgeon may prefer to spend their time in the operating room, but they must have an active outpatient clinic where they evaluate the patients pre- and post-operatively. A family physician, however, will spend most of their time with clinic visits, but may round on their patients when hospitalized.

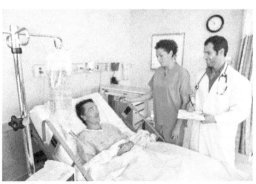
© Tyler Olson, 2014. Used under license fron Shutterstock, Inc.

A day in the clinic will depend on the busyness of the physician's practice. Normally, the physician will arrive before clinic starts, which is often before 8:00 a.m. The number of clinic patients will be highly variable depending on the clinic, the specialty, and whether the patient is new or established in the clinic. Some clinics may only involve four to five patients in a half-day while others may have 15 patients in a half-day. Even though patients have a chief complaint associated with the appointment, things can change when they see the physician. Other issues may be explored and emergencies may arise as well. For example, an obstetrics patient may come in for a fifteen-minute check-up to find that she is fully dilated and needs to go to the delivery room. Keeping a clinic running on time is an art and is often very difficult. Patients typically will be seen on time if they schedule their appointment at the beginning of the day or right after lunch. Provided there were no emergencies, they should be seen on time. Clinic duties would seem to lend themselves to an 8:00 a.m.–5:00 p.m. time frame, however, in addition to seeing patients, a physician must also record their encounter either in the electronic medical record, handwritten notes, or by dictating the encounter. Arranging follow-up and testing may involve more time as well. A thorough clinician is often held up checking labs or other follow-up materials.

If a physician is scheduled to be in the operating room or procedure suite all day, he/she will have a schedule of procedures or surgeries for the day and will conduct their work within that setting. Just like clinic, things are not always predictable and the physician's schedule may be altered due to emergent procedures.

Private Practice vs. Non-Private Practice

Another decision that a physician has to make about their practice is whether to go into private practice working independently, or work for a group, which may be small or large, or directly for a hospital. Government work, such as the Veteran's Administration, is another option as well. Some physicians prefer a military population and choose to work for a Veteran's Administration. These are all personal choices and depend on the type of setting and sometimes the patient population the physician prefers.

Each affords a different type of practice as well as a different lifestyle. There is no right or wrong answer, only preferences for each person. The question is in which type of environment would the physician thrive and which type of environment would he/she find most comfortable. There are pros and cons to every type of practice.

Academic vs. Non-Academic

Some institutions are affiliated with an academic program, but the extent to their involvement can vary. The institution may teach medical students, or train residents, or teach and train students, residents, and fellows. This is dependent upon the agreement that the health care intuition has with the academic institution. For example, a medical school may have many agreements with different hospitals for educating their students to enable their students to participate in rotations at each of those hospital sites. Another type of academic affiliation is that of the medical school owned or partially owned hospital.

All Other Things Considered

The practice of medicine has become so specialized that there is currently a shortage of general practitioners. (http://well.blogs.nytimes.com/2012/12/20 /where-have-all-the-primary-care-doctors-gone/?_r=0)

(http://www.cnbc.com/id/100546118)

This shortage may be for several reasons: students look for something they can fully know and feel comfortable practicing. General medicine is a broad topic and encompasses too much for any one person to know everything. Thus the ambiguity and vast amounts of information are overwhelming to many students. Another reason may be due to a negative perception or stereotype and misconception of primary care training. Some students become detoured from applying to a primary care residency because they are competitive candidates (i.e., high grades and scores) and faculty and fellow students have swayed them to maximize their scores by applying to residencies that are more competitive. In the past, students have actually mentioned that they came into medical school for primary care and that is where their heart is, but they are considering other options because their advisors and classmates thought they were too competitive for primary care. This is a cautionary tale as students should choose a specialty for which they are passionate. Otherwise, they may find themselves in residency again seeking the specialty that makes them happy. Another potential cause for this shortage may be the contrast in compensation between primary care and subspecialties. In reviewing the Money and Medicine Chapter, it is noted that specialties often produce a higher income than primary care fields.

Once a physician has spent time considering their practice and has made some decisions, other factors should be considered. Factors such as geographic location and type of community he/she prefers. The type of practice and chosen specialty will dictate some of this, but consideration should still be given to this. For instance, if the physician is from a small town and truly wants to go back to serve that community (or one similar), then he/she most likely will not want to train in cardiothoracic surgery since this type of practice will be conducted at a larger center that has a certain level of care for critical patients. If the physician would like to be a large part of the community and be "the doctor" that the community turns to, but wants to live in a big city, these two desires are in conflict as this type of doctor is normally found in a small town.

In addition to considering geography, one must consider lifestyle choices. Private practice requires a physician to think about overhead and other aspects that would not be factors for someone that is not self-employed. Some types of practice require more time than others, so seriously considering priorities of life will help when choosing the type of practice that is appropriate for a specific lifestyle.

The practice of medicine is full of choices, choosing a specialty, residency, fellowship, and then subsequently the specifics of their career. The career offers a lot of diversity and requires much decisiveness and awareness of life preferences. However, doctors can change their mind. Physicians have been known to change residencies, go back for further fellowship training, change from private practice to hospital practice, and take on or reduce academic responsibilities. This diversity means that the career of medicine can grow with the physician as their life needs change. Medicine is robust and that means there are and will be endless career opportunities.

Reflections

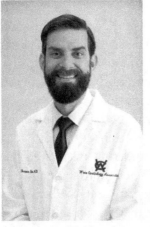

By Shawn J. Skeen, M.D.

I am the first in my family to be a physician and prior to medical school, all of my experiences in clinical practice were spent shadowing. I am a cardiologist and have worked in three very different environments during my relatively short career. I commonly ask medical school applicants during admissions interviews to describe what they believe their practice will look like in 10 years. No detail is too small or insignificant. Don't worry about the specialty, but in general describe the type of town, facility, type of patients, even the color of the carpet in the office if they have envisioned it. Really whatever comes to mind when they close their eyes and envision their future is what I want to know. The options seem limitless, but everyone seems to have at least a primitive vision of what their practice will look like. In fact, when I ask applicants this question and they cannot describe even the simplest vision of their future practice, it makes me wonder if they have thought through being a physician at all. Some of you have had this vision since you were a child. I would have never been able to tell you my specialty if asked that question because I could not have dreamed I would be a cardiologist but I could have described my vision quite clearly. Interestingly, the description I would have given back then of my practice looks very much like the practice I am in today.

During my short career I have worked in several different practice environments. I have worked in a government-operated hospital and clinic, a large academic medical center, and a private practice. Each offers its own special opportunities and obstacles to taking care of patients. These are details that I believe are still too far in your future to consider and can be intimidating. Every year it seems the environment we practice in changes due to economic or regulatory changes beyond our control. You will hear soon enough that the practice of medicine is changing. It always changes and always will. It will also be the most honorable and rewarding career you could ever imagine. It always has been and always will be.

Stop and consider what you want your practice to look like.
Is it a big or small practice?
Do you work alone or do you work with a group of physicians?
Is your ideal practice in a city or small town?
Do you see patients in the hospital, clinic, or both?
Do you like to teach others?
Do your patients travel hundreds of miles to see you or do they live nearby?
Do you work for yourself or do you work for a large company?
Do you want to travel as a part of your practice?
Do you like each day to be different or do you like consistency in what your daily duties are?

These are simple questions and really don't require any significant medical experience to answer. I strongly believe that how you answer these questions now will assist you in determining the type of practice you will be happy in. I also encourage you ask yourself these questions again every 5 years. Your answers may change dramatically or like me not at all, but they will always allow you to reflect on the way you see "your" medical practice. It will allow you to ask yourself, "is the practice I am in now consistent with what I hoped and envisioned." You may be surprised how much your future medical practice will resemble your answers today. I know I am.

I now work in a moderate-sized private practice in a medium-sized city. I no longer teach medical students and residents but I actively teach in the community. I work in both the clinic and the hospital daily. I primarily see patients from within my town but I travel to regional clinics so I can bring my specialty to smaller communities. I have ownership in my practice and it feels very much like running a small business. Each day is very different from the next and my duties may change hour by hour. I love my job and feel very blessed that I asked myself these questions many years ago, and I look forward to asking them throughout my career.

Chapter 11 Worksheet

Why do you want to be a physician?

Which path is right for you?

Answer the following:

Do you like to spend time in the operating room or procedure suite?	**Yes** Need to be in the hospital	**Yes, sometimes** Need some time in the hospital	**No** Clinic
Do you want to be your own boss? Are you OK with the added pressure of owning your own business?	**Yes** Private practice	**Yes, maybe** Consider a small group practice	**No** Hospital employed or group practice
Do you enjoy teaching and/or research?	**Yes** Academic medicine	**Yes, sometimes** Some academics, but it could be incorporated to any type of practice	**No** Avoid academic medicine

Summarize what type of practice you anticipate will be a fit for you.

Is it what you expected? Were there any surprises?

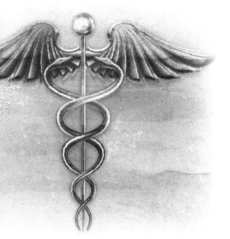

Medicine and Research

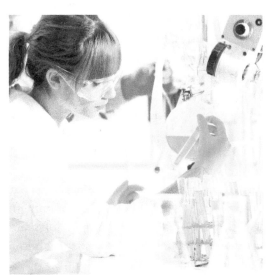

© Matej Kastelic, 2014. Used under license from
Shutterstock, Inc.

What is Research?

If you ever visit a large medical center with a prominent medical school, it is
easy to see with the many elaborate laboratory facilities that research is a significant part of the medical profession. Many premedical students are inspired by
the idea of research and naturally hope to be able to cure major diseases like
cancer or even the common cold. Some students envision large labs with test
tubes, beakers, white rats, and impressive machines that see into the human
body. In truth, this is just a small part of the greater research world of academia
and medicine.

Research is the term we give the process in which we systematically discover new information. It occurs in every aspect of academia, medicine, business, and politics. In the medical professions, it occurs every moment and in
multiple formats ranging from the traditional laboratory to a clinical trial in a
hospital. At a college or university, research is usually being conducted in every
academic department. Nearly every college professor is expected to participate in
some research activity along with his or her graduate students and assistants. It
also seems commonplace to see undergraduate students engaged in research

projects as well. The same is true for the medical profession. Doctor's and other medical professionals are expected to be routinely engaged in research activities.

Why is Research Important to Medicine?

Only a fraction of health care providers actually engage in research activities, but research is highly valued by the medical community. It is impressive what medical doctors and other health care professionals are able to do and what they know in order to manage the many health issues that affect our population. Nonetheless, there is still need for more knowledge that lead to new interventions to support our medical efforts and understanding of disease. Medical personnel need to be employed with the best practices and equipment to help them manage the emerging health issues impacting our global communities.

The new knowledge needed in medicine goes well beyond what can be discovered in the laboratory. New therapies and other medical interventions must be tested in the clinical setting to measure the many other variables that affect the patients. Consequently, medical doctors and other health professionals are needed to engage in medical research to better understand the multitude of health issues that impact our communities and the effectiveness of potential cures and interventions.

The importance of understanding clinical and scientific research extends throughout many facets of the medical field. It is not only important for the researchers, but also for those physicians attempting to integrate such research into their practices. Consequently, many medical students and residents are encouraged to be actively participating in research programs. As the value of medical research is realized, different medical institutions have made attempts to better the situation by offering crash courses in research methodology and interpretation or a mentor in the field. The classes are generally aimed at medical students in their first or second years, residents, and interested physicians. While these classes offer an important foundation of understanding, it does not replace the actual knowledge we get by actually participating in an actual research project. As a result, many medical schools appreciate any research experience an undergraduate student can attain. It is clear that there is a need amongst the medical field to enhance understanding of research methodologies and interpretation. Consequently, many medical schools encourage future applicants to have a demonstrated interest in research during their undergraduate career.

The Association of American Medical Schools (AAMC) has sponsored a website of several undergraduate research programs in the United States **https:// www.aamc.org/members/great/61052/great_summerlinks.html**. This is a great resource for premedical undergraduates in their pursuit of research experiences.

There are several organizations that are committed to medical and health-related research. Premedical students interested in a career as a medical researcher should visit their website to discover future opportunities for their careers.

www.hhmi.org – Howard Hughes Medical Institute
www.nih.gov – National Institutes of Health
www.nsf.gov – National Science Foundation

Bench Research and Medicine

Bench research is likely the classical idea many premedical students have concerning research and medicine. Bench research is typically conducted in a controlled lab environment, usually in the academic fields of biology, chemistry, and biochemistry. In these particular fields of science, bench research is the foundation of new scientific discoveries and critical for the advancement of knowledge in medicine.

Medical knowledge and human physiology are certainly components of the general biological fields. Consequently, there are many bench laboratory techniques that are pertinent to the studies in medicine. Students can easily engage in a multitude of biological topics that will have an impact on our understanding of disease and medicine, such as cell biology, microbiology, virology, genetics, molecular biology, etc. Moreover, biology is a very broad academic field. In biological research, many of the research topics tend to be more generalized and the knowledge is not limited to human interactions or disease. Consequently, students can be engaged in a variety of labs and/or need to develop many different lab techniques to be successful.

There are many venues in which an undergraduate can demonstrate functional lab and research skills in the many academic science fields. Regardless of the research project that you invest your time, there will likely be some knowledge and talents that you can utilize in medicine. For instance, many vaccines and drugs are expressed in plant or yeast platforms. Many biological scientists will be needed to help produce the new drugs and vaccines for future diseases. Moreover, understanding the physiological and anatomical features of other species will always have some benefit in understanding our own physiology. Additionally, many biological research labs will help you become proficient in using instruments such as microscopes and other observational equipment.

Much like the academic field of biology, there are many opportunities for the field of medicine to be advanced through bench research in chemistry and biochemistry. In this type of research, the nature of the work is generally confined to laboratories and the ideas are focused on the chemical processes. In medicine, this will have a significant impact on the general metabolism of the human body as well as cell metabolism. Moreover, research in chemistry and biochemistry help us to better understand genetics and DNA expression. The many research projects conducted in the fields of chemistry and biochemistry are certainly cutting-edge and will have a significant impact on medicine in the future. If you enjoy working in the biochemistry/chemistry laboratories, there will be many opportunities for you to participate in meaningful research.

Translational Research and Medicine

Translation and bench research are very similar and can easily be confused. Typically, a traditional bench researcher in science will simply focus on researching a specific biological or chemical process. In translational research, this biological or chemical process will be applied to a physiological/living system. In medicine, this can take place in many different platforms: plant, animal, cellular, or human physiology. So if a chemist discovers a process to create a new drug, they will likely work with a translational researcher to see how it may be applied to a physiological system.

Much like bench research, translational research is also confined to a controlled laboratory setting, but most translation research projects will use animals or plants to conduct the research. This is especially important in the development of new therapies or drugs that are being tested for potential medical benefits. The animals or plants are used to measure the effectiveness of new therapies/drugs, while providing opportunities to observe and discover other physiological activities or side effects. Before any new drug can be used on humans for medical benefits, it has to be tested in a variety of animals and/or plants.

Translational research projects will be ideal for those individuals that enjoy working in a laboratory setting, but want to focus on issues that apply to physiological outcomes. Moreover, a translational researcher should be comfortable working with a variety of animals and have a significant interest and background in human and animal physiology.

Clinical Research and Medicine

Most medical doctors will likely spend most of their time and effort participating in clinical research. Clinical research is focused on discovering/measuring the effectiveness of new treatments, drugs, and protocols in health care. As can be determined by its name, clinical research is generally conducted in a clinical or hospital setting. The research is generally focused on outcomes in patient care, but there are certainly a wide variety of topics and issues that can be investigated. Clinical research can involve the measurement of new surgical techniques, pharmaceutical trials, and general patient satisfaction. Clinical research is necessary to apply the knowledge gained from bench and translational research programs.

Since clinical research is not performed in a lab like bench and translational research, physicians and the other medical researchers do not generally need expensive equipment to conduct their research projects. Although, access to patients and creating a controlled environment does present other challenges to conducting a successful research project. Moreover, there are many ethical issues that have to be addressed since most clinical research involves patients. Consequently, many medical researchers work with Institutional Review Boards (IRB) to ensure they are conducting safe and ethical research. Most colleges and universities support their own IRBs and students can learn more about medical research ethics at www.citiprogram.org.

Since many future physicians will be engaged in clinical research, premedical students will certainly benefit from exposure to clinical research programs. Premedical students will have to be intentional in seeking these opportunities since they do not readily exist in most college science departments. If you are interested in participating in clinical research programs, you will have to seek opportunities at medical schools or other large medical centers. At times, individual physicians or other health care professionals may be engaged in clinical research as well.

Public Health Research and Medicine

Public health research is an integral part of the health care system. Public health is an academic field that has several distinct divisions: epidemiology, community health, environmental health, global health, public policy, health economics, and occupational health. All of these branches of public health utilize research to support the delivery of health care. Unlike clinical research, most public health research projects are concerned with prevalence of disease, overall health outcomes, and the general health of a specific population. This information is vital for other medical researchers and health care professionals in general. As a consequence of public health research, we can direct appropriate resources and research efforts to address emerging health issues. There are many opportunities for medical personnel and students to participate in public health research studies. The cost of public health research can be relatively inexpensive and there is public access to much of the data, however, it does require a functional background in statistics and/or biostatistics.

Selecting a Research Project

There are so many different aspects to medical research that it can be very challenging for an undergraduate premedical student to determine what is the best research project for them. Moreover, the research opportunities on most college campuses are limited, especially for undergraduate students. Nevertheless, there is little value for a student to participate in a research project that they have little intellectual or personal interest in investigating. Moreover, quality research demands a great deal of personal effort and time, so premedical students need to be careful before joining a lab or initiating a research project.

There are several other variables that a student researcher needs to address as well. Before starting a research project, the researcher needs to determine what resources will be needed to conduct the study. If the population or lab materials are not available, there is little chance for the study to be successful. For most undergraduates, the faculty research mentors that are available to them limit their ability to engage in any specific project. Nevertheless, they can begin their research efforts by simply engaging in the literature of their desired topic.

To begin, researchers and premedical students can visit several websites to expand and explore a variety of medical topics. A free website called Medical Subject Headings (MeSH) can be used to properly define multiple medical topics **http://www.ncbi.nlm.nih.gov/mesh**. MeSH will also link research to other research websites like PubMed (**http://www.ncbi.nlm.nih.gov/pubmed/**) that will allow them to search for a multitude of medical journals and other research articles. Moreover, many college/university library systems will provide undergraduates with access to other medical databases (**http://www.nlm.nih.gov/bsd/pmresources.html#**) that will be helpful in supporting any research efforts.

Undergraduates should begin to immerse themselves in research by exploring medical research databases. Your college librarians can be a great resource to navigating the many databases, but we have included some general tips on using the databases.

How to use databases like PubMed and Web of Science:

- Search for articles based on topic, author, journal, year of publication, or key words in title and any combination.
- Sort results by different filters:
  - "By Publication Date" will show you the most recent articles in a field.
  - "By Times Cited" will show you the most commonly cited, which are usually the most important articles in the field.
- Group all works by one particular author. This is helpful when beginning your review and looking for articles to include in your search.
- Create a marked list. A marked list will allow you to tag all interesting articles and store them in one place. You can then email this to yourself, print it out, or send it to a bibliography maker.
- Create citation alerts that email you whenever a related article is published.
- Create citation map. This tool shows the citation history and use of the article in question.

Getting Ready for Research:

1. Make your own database (Web of Science/PubMed) account.
2. First, search by subject keywords to find the most recent and the most cited articles in your field.
3. Use the bibliography of the most cited articles to find additional resources for your project.
4. Create a citation alert for most pertinent articles.
5. REMEMBER! Save all articles to bibliography maker as you go!

Reading Medical Research Literature

Reading and finding medical research literature can be very difficult for many students. Research literature is generally very dense and it is usually written for other experts in medicine/science. With limited research or medical background, it will be challenging to interpret the findings or discussion presented in the literature. Consequently, undergraduate premedical students will need to engage in the appropriate coursework and seek the support of knowledgeable mentors to assist in their initial efforts in reading medical literature.

Summary Overview

Research is certainly a vital component of the medical professions and necessary in order to discover new therapies and treatments that will cure diseases and alleviate suffering; however, not every premedical student has to be a researcher. If you find a research project or topic that genuinely inspires and excites your intellectual interests, then you will likely be a successful researcher. On the other hand, if the research project does not hold your interests, then you may want to carefully discern whether or not you want to spend a lifetime pursuing it.

Research is not summer activity or something to simply add to your resume. It should be a result of your intellectual curiosity and a desire to pursue scholarly activities. To perform good research, you will have to invest a great deal of time and effort to learn the appropriate techniques and maybe develop new ones in order to attain and interpret the data. Both laboratory and clinical research are intensive and at times arduous activities, but it certainly has the potential to positively affect many lives and for some it could change the world. Reflect carefully about your intellectual passions and be diligent in your efforts to participate in research. Medicine needs good researchers as much as it needs good and compassionate health care providers.

Undergraduate Reflections on Research

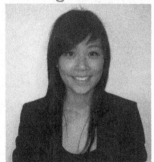

By Vivian P. Nguyen
Baylor University Undergraduate Student, 2010–2014

The work I had done for my Honors Thesis helped me grow and realize a number of things. I gained an appreciation and respect for research after having to learn the methods and go through each arduous step in the process.

I began working on my thesis in the spring of my sophomore year, so it has been a work in progress for nearly two years. During this period, I felt and still continue to feel that learning to do research is like learning a new language, and it took a while before I got the hang of the idea. It was difficult for me to do something entirely out of my comfort zone. At the start, I had no idea how to do a literature review or how to come up with a questionnaire for my study. Just the thought of analyzing data was extremely nebulous to me. Many times, I almost felt like it was all a daze because it was so different from the usual, out-of-the-textbook stuff. Learning an answer to a question is one thing, but searching for the answer is entirely another.

I think that having a resourceful, patient, and encouraging mentor was what helped me most. There were a lot of times throughout the research process, mainly during the data entry and analysis part, when I felt frustrated and/or at a loss because things did not go the way we had expected or we did not find the relationships/ outcomes we had hoped to find.

I learned, however, that it was all just a part of research. Research is messy because you adjust as you go along and you need to rely on yourself and your research team. Naturally, there would be errors—whether human, random, or systematic—and unexpected problems would occur along the way. There was one point when I was about to analyze my data only to discover that half of it was missing because it was skipped somehow when our team was entering it. I also had to throw out a number of variables simply because there were inconsistencies in how our information was gathered. Challenges such as these were frustrating to me but helped me to gain patience for uncertainty as well as a newfound perspective on medicine.

(continued)

Undergraduate Reflections on Research *(continued)*

Medicine, like research, has specific protocol and methodology, but not everything is predictable and the outcome isn't always easily reached. Sometimes complications arise, and creativity and critical thinking are required to solve problems within problems. In other words, you have to be willing to deal with uncertainty on multiple levels. As I'm nearing the stages of completing my thesis, I realize that research served as a valuable experience for me because it complements my desire to become a medical doctor. © Kendall Hunt Publishing Company.

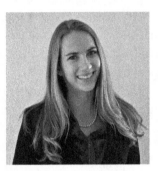

By Kelli Hicks
Baylor University Undergraduate Student, 2010–2014

I switched off the lights and peered into the microscope to carefully count the nuclei speckled with Green Fluorescence Protein and recorded the numbers on my data sheet. "Well," I thought to myself, "this gene also doesn't play a role in protein tagging." What was the pathway? How exactly did the cell go about tagging a protein to signal the rest of the cell to destroy it? I had access to a multitude of resources and equipment in this lab, but none of it could give me these answers. I was responsible for putting together this puzzle by myself. This challenge and these questions formed a large part of my scholastic experience and as a natural questioner and problem solver, I thrived in the opportunity to find the answers and explore this novel avenue.

As a freshman, I invested myself in diligently experimenting on the model organism *Caenorhabditis elegans*. After learning the basic mechanics and procedures of the lab, my mentor helped me compose an experiment, which assumed knowledge far beyond my current academic level. I pored over journal articles and textbooks and earnestly questioned both my mentor and the graduate students in the lab in order to wholly understand and learn the new concepts. During my sophomore year, I gained almost complete autonomy to design and to direct my own experiment. In designing experiments, reading current literature, and writing about my results, I learned to think creatively and cultivated my ability to be flexible in adjusting experiments.

It is this questioning and challenging environment that also draws me into the medical field. Medicine, like research, often has no clear-cut answer and one must rely upon previous experience and problem-solving abilities to find the best solution.

© Kendall Hunt Publishing Company

Research in Medicine Reflection

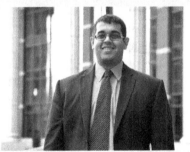

By Kevin P. Shah
Baylor College of Medicine, Class of 2019

I remember in high school when I used to think that doing research meant sitting in a lab and staring at cell specimens under a microscope all day. Little did I know that this image barely brushed the surface of what medical research actually entails. Each one of us, whether we know it or not, have engaged in research throughout our lives. It may have been determining the fastest route to a specific destination, finding the most effective way to study for a class, or even investigating which ingredients make the perfect sandwich.

In classes and lectures, we are always learning about what is known in the world. Research is the one opportunity we have to make a difference by exploring and discovering the unknown. It is what allows medicine to advance and evolve through new and innovative technologies, therapeutic interventions, and improved clinical guidelines for patient care. A world without research is unimaginable. Who knows what the practice of medicine would be like today without research? It is quite possible that we would still be engaging in absurd medical practices such as bloodletting or drinking radioactive water to cure disease.

Unlike many of the projects and assignments we receive in school, research can often be unstructured and fragmented. There will be times, as a researcher, where you don't know exactly what the next step will be. There will be times that you get completely unexpected results. There will be times you simply just fail. At the end of the day, what ultimately shapes your success in research is your ability to take initiative and overcome these adversities.

Throughout my undergraduate career, I had the opportunity to engage in clinical and operational research within cancer care and behavioral health. If there is one thing I have learned from these experiences, it is the importance of persistence and perseverance. At any given time, research can either be the most rewarding or the most frustrating experience you have had. Nonetheless, it serves a purpose in teaching you a skillset that cannot be taught in the classroom: the ability to think critically and solve problems in a real-world setting. This particular set of skills requires hands-on learning through the practice of research.

As a researcher, you will be called upon to question everything and stop at nothing. You will be faced with thought-provoking questions such as "how can I improve upon a clinical workflow process that has been in place for decades?" or "how can we disseminate findings of new technologies and interventions to physicians worldwide in a timely manner?" These questions, unlike others you may have tackled before, do not necessarily have a right answer. They definitely do not have a simple one. However, it is up to you to rise to the challenge and find a solution to these daunting, yet pivotal questions.

As I reflect back upon my exposure to research, I realize how instrumental it has been in impacting my future career goals and aspirations. A mentor once described research to me as an avenue to impact the lives of patients on a global scale. He said, "by treating patients, you can only help a set number of people in a single day, but through research, the number of people you can help has no limits."

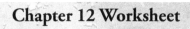

Chapter 12 Worksheet
Research

What type of research is being conducted at the top two medical schools you selected in Chapter 2?

1)

2)

What type of research do you find most interesting (Bench, Translational, Clinical)?

Is there a specific medical topic/issue that you would like to research?

Are you interested in pursuing a dual degree (PhD, MPH, MBA, MS) along with your medical education? If so, what would be your ideal joint graduate program and what benefits will it have for your future?

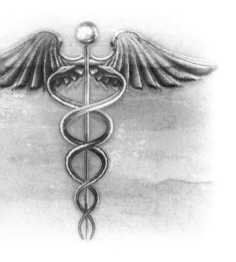

Chapter 13
Money and Medicine

Medicine is certainly a complex industry and is greatly misunderstood by those of us that receive medical care and the many students seeking to join the health care professions. In this chapter, Dr. William Neilson, former Vice President of the BSA Health System, discusses in detail the many venues in which money affects the delivery of health care and the practice of medicine in the United States.

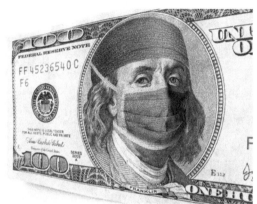

© Richardo Reitmeyer, 2014. Used under license from Shutterstock, Inc.

Cost of Medical Education

The data discussed in this section is drawn from the AAMC publication *Physician Education Debt and the Cost to Attend Medical School 2012 Update* by James "Jay" Youngclaus and Julie A. Fresne. (https://www.aamc.org/download /328322/data/statedebtreport.pdf).

Based upon the American Association of Medical Colleges (AAMC) 2012 data, the average in-state four-year cost of attendance (tuition, fees, and living expenses) is $228,200. This overwhelming cost is funded by a combination of scholarships and loans for about 86% of all medical students. The likelihood of obtaining a scholarship is dependent upon the type of medical school attended with private schools having significantly more scholarship opportunities than public schools. Of course, the four-year private medical school cost of attendance ($275,305) is much greater than that for public schools ($196,661).

As demonstrated in the graph on the next page, the four-year cost of attendance of medical school has significantly increased in the past decade. Because the cost of medical school is so great and because it is impractical to work during medical school, it is uncommon for anyone to attend without borrowing significant amounts of money or receiving a large scholarship or grant. MD/PhD students have a greater chance of having tuition fully covered

Figure 13-1. Median 4-year cost of attendance (COA) and education debt of indebted medical school graduates, 2000–2012 (In constant 2012 dollars)

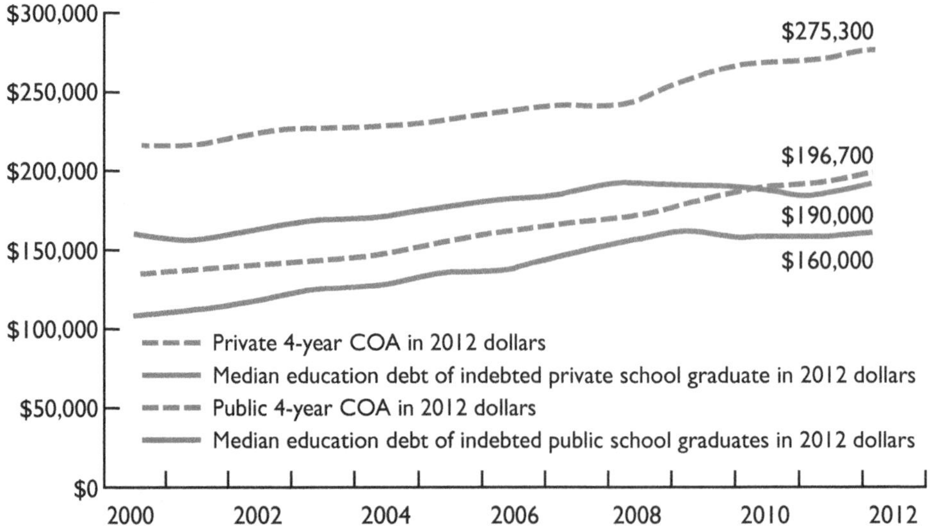

Source: AAMC Graduation Questionnaire (GQ) and Tuition and Student Fees Survey (TSF).

From, *Physician Education Debt and the Cost to Attend Medical School*, by the Association of American Medical Colleges. Copyright © 2013 by the Association of American Medical Colleges. Reprinted by permission.

by grants or scholarships. Full scholarships are unusual in other circumstances; however, about 60% of students have some form of scholarship assistance, which averages <$20,000 for four years.

The average medical school educational debt was $170,000 in 2012. As would be expected, the debt is greater for those attending private medical schools than for those attending public medical schools. Debt levels are expected to increase 5–6% per year based upon historical trends.

Currently, medical students can borrow up to $40,500 annually through the Stafford Loan program; however, interest begins to accrue upon borrowing the money. Interest rates are floating and repayment provisions vary depending upon the choice of the student. It is possible to delay repayment until after residency, but interest accrues during residency if this option is chosen. The AAMC has a loan calculator on its website that will assist students in choosing repayment options.

Several programs exist for loan forgiveness. The National Health Service Corps has a repayment program that repays up to $60,000 for a two-year commitment to work in a medically underserved area as a primary care provider. In addition, the Public Service Loan Forgiveness Program (PSLF) cancels remaining debt for those working for a non-profit entity or the government.

Practice Income

Eventually, physicians complete medical school and begin to generate income. Physician incomes are significant and vary widely depending upon specialty. Medscape performs an annual compensation survey, which can be reviewed at http://www.medscape.com/features/slideshow/compensation/2013/public?src=

wnl_edit_specol&uac=122617BX. This survey suggests a range of average compensation from $170,000 to $405,000 depending upon specialty. Obviously, there are outliers in both the high and low ends of the spectrum. Even the "lowest paid" physicians will earn far more money than the average American; it is sobering to recall that the median annual salary in the United States in 2010 was $26,363.20. (Jeremy M. Blumberg, MD. *Considering Life before Lifestyle. JAMA.* 2012; 307(20):2159–2160. doi: 10.1001/jama.2012.4522)

Figure 13-2.

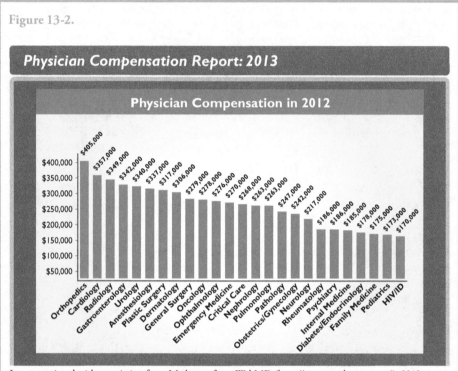

Physician Compensation Report: 2013

Physician Compensation in 2012

Image reprinted with permission from Medscape from WebMD (http://www.medscape.com/), 2013, available at: http://www.medscape.com/features/slideshow/compensation/2013/public.

Income varies based upon practice setting. Historically, the practice of medicine was a "cottage industry" with most physicians in a solo or small group practice. This has changed dramatically in recent years and currently the majority of physicians are "employed" upon finishing residency. "Employed" is a non-specific term and may range from academic positions to hospital employment to employment by a large group. Salaries vary dramatically depending upon the source of employment, perceived need, and specialty. A hospital that can demonstrate significant need for a specific specialty is likely willing to arrange student loan repayment over the course of a long-term contract.

Figure 13-3.

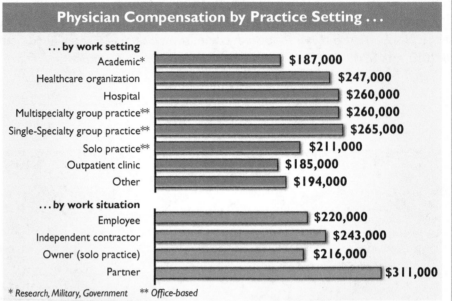

Image reprinted with permission from Medscape from WebMD (http://www.medscape.com/), 2013, available at: http://www.medscape.com/features/slideshow/compensation/2013/public.

Most practicing physicians do not realize that hospitals cannot compensate physicians above "fair market value (FMV)." The assessment of fair market value must include all compensation and ideally be performed by a third party. Both the physician and the hospital are at risk of violating federal law if compensation is deemed to be excessive.

There are advantages and disadvantages for each practice setting. The key advantage to solo (or small group) practice is autonomy; however, this is likely more than offset by the responsibilities of running the practice. The physician in a small practice must manage finances, personnel, pension plans, health insurance, collections, etc. Physicians typically have no training in any of these areas and are busy caring for patients; therefore, as practice has become more complex, physicians have sought to join larger organizations that can afford to hire practice management professionals.

There are multiple advantages to large group practice and one distinct disadvantage. The advantages are obvious: the group can afford to hire a professional practice administrator to allow the physicians to practice medicine without worrying about the details of making the practice function. Large groups also have financial stability and are able to generate favorable terms with insurance companies because of their size. The significant potential disadvantage is the loss of autonomy. Most physician groups are dysfunctional democracies. The partners will rarely vote to override the desires of a vocal minority, and, therefore, the group is unable to make difficult decisions. In addition, the practice of medicine requires a sense of camaraderie, which may be difficult to form in larger groups.

Hospital employment is even more complex. In Texas, the law prohibits the corporate practice of medicine, which means that, in general, hospitals cannot employ physicians. Hospitals deal with this problem by creating a physician-governed entity called a Non-profit Healthcare Corporation under section 501.A of the tax code. Such entities are also called 501(a)s and, although governed by physicians, are likely controlled indirectly and financially by the "member" hospital. As mentioned above, physician compensation must be in compliance with federal law and therefore FMV.

Academic medicine also has distinct advantages and disadvantages. Historically, those in academic practice have lower incomes than those in private practice. In an era of increasing austerity, medical schools have come to rely progressively on a portion of practice income (the Dean's tax) to fund operations. Academic practice is multi-faceted as the practitioner likely has a private practice, a teaching service, and research responsibilities. The advantage is the opportunity to teach and the fact that residents perform many of the duties needed to care for the sick. Current Medicare and Medicaid regulations require the presence of the attending during critical parts of patient care.

Employed physician compensation is typically negotiated and based upon the RVU system noted below. This is important, as it allows more productive physicians to be more highly compensated. The risk to the health care system involves incentivizing physicians to do more procedures.

Management of a medical practice is extremely complicated. Overhead may be as high as 40–50% of collections and collection of bad debt is problematic, because many physicians do not wish to pursue collections by legal means. It is not unusual to have two support personnel (or more) per physician, which means that a single physician's collections may be the main source of income for three families. Practice expenses include: rent or mortgage payments, costs of recruiting physicians or nurses, utilities, health insurance, malpractice insurance, retirement plans for employees and physicians, furnishing an office, maintenance, computer hardware, software for billing and electronic medical records, phone lines, high-speed Internet connections, continuing medical education expenses, payroll taxes, legal fees, etc. The list seems endless. An example of a spreadsheet (courtesy of Eileen Harpole, Director of BSA Clinics) utilized to create a practice pro forma is in the chart on the next page:

Project Name:		Proforma Template					
Anticipated Start Date:	TBD						

	Year 1	Year 2	Year 3	Year 4	Year 5	Year 6	
Gross Revenue							
IP Revenue	-	-	-	-	-	-	Automatic Calculation based on IP Volumes and IP Revenue/Unit
OP Revenue	-	-	-	-	-	-	Automatic Calculation based on OP Volumes and OP Revenue/Unit
Total Gross Revenue	-	-	-	-	-	-	Automatic Calculation
Revenue Deductions							
Charity	-	-	-	-	-	-	Automatic Calculation based on Charity %
Other Contractuals	-	-	-	-	-	-	Automatic Calculation based on Other Rev Deduction %
Total Revenue Deductions	-	-	-	-	-	-	Automatic Calculation
Net Patient Service Revenue	-	-	-	-	-	-	Automatic Calculation
Total Revenue	-	-	-	-	-	-	Automatic Calculation
Operating Expenses							
Employee Salary & Wages		-	-	-	-	-	Enter FY 11 only, the rest automatically calculates
Employee Benefits		-	-	-	-	-	Automatic Calculation
Contract Labor	-	-	-	-	-	-	Enter FY 11 only, the rest automatically calculates
Professional Fees		-	-	-	-	-	Enter FY 11 only, the rest automatically calculates
Supplies		-	-	-	-	-	Enter FY 11 only, the rest automatically calculates
Pharmaceuticals		-	-	-	-	-	Enter FY 11 only, the rest automatically calculates
Purchased Services		-	-	-	-	-	Enter FY 11 only, the rest automatically calculates
Depreciation & Amortization	-	-	-	-	-	-	Automatic Calculation
Other Expense		-	-	-	-	-	Enter FY 11 only, the rest automatically calculates
Bad Debt	-	-	-	-	-	-	Automatic Calculation
Total Operating Expenses	-	-	-	-	-	-	Automatic Calculation
Income From Operations	$ -	$ -	$ -	$ -	$ -	$ -	

IP Data:							
Patient Days		-	-	-	-	-	Automatic Calculation
Discharges (# of Patients)		-	-	-	-	-	Enter INCREMENTAL Data Here
ALOS	-	-	-	-	-	-	Based on BSA FY 11 Budget. Change if Needed
IP Volume Growth Rate		3.00%	3.00%	3.00%	3.00%	3.00%	Enter Rev/Unit (Entire Hospital Stay) in FY 11
IP Rev/Unit (For Entire Hospital Stay)	$ -	$ -	$ -	$ -	$ -		Enter Rev/Unit (Entire Hospital Stay) in FY 11
Inflation Rate		4.00%	4.00%	4.00%	4.00%	4.00%	

OP Data:							
OP Visits		-	-	-	-	-	Enter INCREMENTAL Data Here
OP Volume Growth Rate		3.00%	3.00%	3.00%	3.00%	3.00%	
OP Rev/Unit (For Entire Hospital Visit)	$ -	$ -	$ -	$ -	$ -		Enter Rev/Unit (Entire Hospital Stay) in FY 11
Inflation Rate		4.00%	4.00%	4.00%	4.00%	4.00%	

Revenue Deductions:							
Charity	6.93%	6.93%	6.93%	6.93%	6.93%	6.93%	Based on previous year Budget: Charity as a % of Gross
Other Deductions	63.15%	63.15%	63.15%	63.15%	63.15%	63.15%	Based on previous year Budget: All Other Deductions as a % of Gross

Other Expense Data Inflation %:							
Employee Salary & Wages		3.00%	3.00%	3.00%	3.00%	3.00%	Based on previous year Budget
Employee Benefits	22.13%	22.13%	22.13%	22.13%	22.13%	22.13%	Based on previous year Budget
Contract Labor		3.00%	3.00%	3.00%	3.00%	3.00%	Based on previous year Budget
Professional Fees		3.00%	3.00%	3.00%	3.00%	3.00%	Based on previous year Budget
Supplies		3.00%	3.00%	3.00%	3.00%	3.00%	Based on previous year Budget
Pharmaceuticals		3.00%	3.00%	3.00%	3.00%	3.00%	Based on previous year Budget
Purchased Services		3.00%	3.00%	3.00%	3.00%	3.00%	Based on previous year Budget
Other Expense		3.00%	3.00%	3.00%	3.00%	3.00%	Based on previous year Budget
Bad Debt	2.84%	2.84%	2.84%	2.84%	2.84%	2.84%	Based on previous year Budget: Bad Debt as a % of Net

FTE's							
Employed Hours	-	-	-	-	-	-	Automatic Calculation
Contract Labor Hours	-	-	-	-	-	-	Automatic Calculation
Employed FTE's							Enter Incremental FTE's Here
Contract Labor FTE's							Enter Incremental FTE's Here
Employed AHWR	$ -	$ -	$ -	$ -	$ -	$ -	Automatic Calculation
Contract AWHR	$ -	$ -	$ -	$ -	$ -	$ -	Automatic Calculation

Capital:		
FFE		Enter Data Here
Expected Useful Life (in years)		Enter Data Here
Expected Date of Purchase		Enter Data Here

Financial Assessment:	1 Year	2 Years	3 Years	4 Years	5 Years	6 Years
Return on Investment	0.00%	0.00%	0.00%	0.00%	0.00%	0.00%

6-Year Net Present Value $0.00   Discount Rate   10%
*Assume capital expenditure at beginning of fiscal year and net operating income at end of fiscal year.

Internal Rate of Return	Not Applicable	Not Applicable	Not Applicable	Not Applicable	Not Applicable	Not Applicable

IRR Hurdle Rate   6.50%   Is final IRR greater than the hurdle rate?   No

Reprinted by permission of BSA Physicians Group, Inc.

Beyond generating enough income to cover the basic costs of practice, there are countless negotiations and legal issues to consider. The most important negotiations are typically those with health insurance companies in the determination of reimbursement. Physicians are reimbursed based upon CPT (current procedural terminology) codes and the reimbursement amount is frequently only marginally related to the complexity or cost of patient care. Legal issues which must be considered include following employment laws, compliance with the ADA, and basic understanding of Stark laws (which will be considered briefly later in the chapter).

Retirement plans are exceedingly complex legal entities. Many physicians do not provide retirement for their employees, but this decision limits the kinds of retirement plans that a practice can utilize. Most large groups of doctors provide at least a 401K plan and provide matching funds to increase employee participation. Under such arrangements, most doctors can contribute in the range of $30,000 of pre-tax income annually, but they also contribute significantly to employee accounts.

Malpractice premiums are a major contributor to practice overhead. Employed physicians do not have to arrange malpractice coverage. Obviously, physicians in solo or small practices must negotiate and buy malpractice insurance. In Texas, with the passage of tort reform, the annual premiums have dropped by as much as 50%. Prior to tort reform, there were only two malpractice carriers left in Texas, which drastically limited competition. Currently, there are many carriers with varying stability and cost structures. There are two basic types of malpractice insurance: occurrence and claims made. Both claims made and occurrence policies are renewed annually. Occurrence policies cover the insured in perpetuity for actions that occurred while the policy was in effect. As a result, occurrence policies are more expensive and have a relatively stable annual premium. Claims made policies cover the insured for acts that occur during the year of coverage but only if a claim is made during that year. Coverage for succeeding years must be purchased from the same company in order to maintain coverage for prior years; therefore, the annual premium increases for four to five years before stabilizing. If the physician opts to change insurers, "tail" coverage (which provides insurance for the prior years in perpetuity) must be purchased from the existing company or "nose or prior acts" coverage (which picks up coverage for years insured by the prior company) must be purchased from the new company. There are also dramatic differences upon retirement. Because occurrence policies cover the insured in perpetuity, the retiring physician simply stops paying premiums upon retirement. In order to have coverage after retirement, those with claims made policies must buy a tail policy that is typically about 200% of the last year's premium. Many policies will provide tail coverage free of charge if the retiring physician is over 55 and has been insured by the company for five years.

The following tables show the specialty class and demonstrate the drastic differences in malpractice premiums depending upon specialty and the differences between claims made and occurrence policies. There are also variations depending upon regional differences in the likelihood of being sued.

Class	Specialty
I	Dermatology, Allergy, Psychiatry
II	Internal Medicine, Oncology, Anesthesiology
III	Pulmonology, Gastroenterology, Non-invasive Cardiology
IV	ENT, Urology, Neurology

continued

Class	Specialty
V	Hand Surgery, Emergency Medicine, Gynecology, Orthopedic Surgery
VI	OB/GYN, Cardiovascular Surgery, Vascular Surgery, General Surgery
VII	Trauma Surgery
VIII	Bariatric Surgery, Neurosurgery

Dallas Area $1,000,000/$3,000,000
($1,000,000 per event; $3,000,000 per year)

Class	Claims Made Year 0	Claims Made Year 1	Claims Made Year 2	Claims Made Year 3 +	Occurrence
I	~$3,700	~$5,500	~$9,000	~$10,500	~$11,000/yr
II	~$5,500	~$8,000	~$13,000	~$15,500	~$16,000/yr
III	~$7,000	~$10,000	~$17,000	~$20,000	~$28,500/yr
IV	~$9,500	~$14,000	~$23,000	~$27,500	~$28,500/yr
V	~$12,500	~$18,000	~$30,500	~$36,000	~$37,000/yr
VI	~$18,500	~$27,000	~$44,000	~$52,500	~$53,000/yr
VII	~$22,250	~$32,500	~$54,000	~$63,500	~$65,300/yr
VIII	~$33,000	~$48,000	~$80,000	~$94,500	~$97,000/yr

McAllen Area $1,000,000/$3,000,000

Class	Claims Made Year 0	Claims Made Year 1	Claims Made Year 2	Claims Made Year 3+	Occurrence
I	~$6,200	~$9,000	~$15,000	~$17,750	~$18,000
II	~$9,200	~$13,250	~$22,000	~$26,250	~$26,750
III	~$12,000	~$17,000	~$28,500	~$33,500	~$34,500
IV	~$16,000	~$23,500	~$39,250	~$46,250	~$47,500
V	~$21,000	~$30,500	~$51,000	~$60,600	~$62,000
VI	~$32,000	~$34,000	~$75,000	~$89,500	~$91,750
VII	~$37,400	~$54,250	~$90,500	~$107,000	~$109,500
VIII	~$55,500	~$80,500	~$134,500	~$158,500	~$162,500

(The above data is courtesy of Neely, Craig, and Walton Insurance of Amarillo, TX. The insurance company name has been redacted at their request.)

Computer systems are a major financial cost of every practice. There are multiple vendors selling practice management systems and the various systems vary in cost and features. In theory, all EMR systems can communicate with one another based upon HL7 (Health Level 7), which is an entity that creates standards allowing transfer of health information. Both the ARRA and HITECH laws require HL7 compatibility. Unfortunately, on a practical level, HL7 is not adequate to allow communication between different EMRs (such as hospital to physician's office). This requires the creation of expensive computer interfaces, which each may cost as much as $20,000/year to maintain and must be modified with each release of new software. A decision regarding which system to purchase is of critical importance and most practices drop drastically in productivity upon the change from paper to EMR. The ARRA provides up to $44,000/physician when the practice achieves "meaningful use" criteria. Whether or not EMRs save money or improve patient care is very controversial. Further complexity is added with the recognition that not all EMRs are also adequate for billing purposes.

The decision to join a group practice is not as simple as simply signing up and going to work. Each practice will have a different method of dividing income and most practices have some sort of "buy in" provision wherein new partners must buy a portion of the practice assets before they can share profits of the practice. Depending upon the philosophy of the practice, the buy in amount may be quite large—possibly >$100,000. It behooves the young physician to carefully assess practice opportunities to determine what the ultimate expenses might be to join a practice.

It is not necessarily easy to leave a practice once joined. Most employed physicians (whether by a group or hospital) sign a "non-compete" in their employment contract. Such clauses are intended to discourage leaving employment and to compensate the employer for lost income if the physician does leave. In Texas, non-compete clauses are not enforceable unless they are financially reasonable. In the eyes of the state of Texas, the contract should not be able to deprive the patient of his physician; however, the state does allow enforcement of significant financial penalties for leaving employment and staying in the area. For example, a non-compete clause might require payment to the employer that would compensate the employer for the expenses of starting the physician's practice and even hiring a replacement. Such a non-compete provision could easily be in six digits. Regardless of the cost of a non-compete, the employer has no authority to disrupt the doctor patient relationship and the physician can "keep" his patients if the patients so desire.

Stark laws are federal laws named after Pete Stark, (D-CA), which intend to limit physician self-referral and outlaw many financial relationships between hospitals and physicians. The regulated financial relationships include physician employment, compensation to physicians for services provided by hospitals, and ancillary services provided in physician offices. For example, physicians must disclose to patients ownership in diagnostic imaging centers or labs. Hospitals must ensure that all financial transactions with physicians (compensation, partnerships, acquisitions) meet the test of fair market value. Physicians are also prohibited from accepting kickbacks that involve accepting funds for referrals. Many doctors simply assume that it is reasonable to accept remuneration for sending patients to a specific hospital; however, such an arrangement would clearly represent a kickback under the law. Any incentive provided to physicians to encourage referral to a hospital is likely a violation of the law. Such issues become more complicated when a physician accepts compensation for emergency room call. Call compensation has become commonplace; however, compensation above FMV could be a violation of Stark and/or anti-kickback laws. Obviously, the physician in solo practice must seek legal counsel before entering into any financial relationship with a hospital.

Medicare/Medicaid and Insurance Companies

Physician compensation is based upon CPT codes, which describe patient encounters or procedures done by the physician upon the patient. Historically, such compensation was based upon "usual and customary" payments, which were based upon tradition and not science. Everything began to change rather dramatically with the landmark publication *Results and Policy Implications of the Resource-Based Relative-Value Study* (William C. Hsiao, PhD, Peter Braun, MD, Daniel Dunn, PhD, Edmund R. Becker, PhD, Margaret DeNicola, MPH, and Thomas R. Ketcham, MPH, *N Engl J Med* 319 [1988]: 881–888 September 29, 1988 doi:10.1056/NEJM198809293191330).

This article resulted in the transformation of physician compensation by linking physician work across specialties. The goal was to create a logical system for determining the amount of work, practice cost, and opportunity cost for each CPT code. The codes are then assigned a value termed RVU (relative value unit). As might be expected, the original concept has been modified and subject to political pressures. Currently, annual meetings of the Specialty Society Relative Value Scale Update Committee (RUC) update the RVUs. The RVU for a given code varies geographically to account for malpractice costs and practice expenses. The current formula is

Medicare PFS Payment Rates Formula

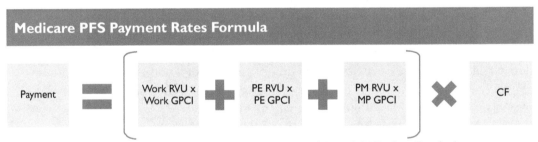

https://www.cms.gov/Outreach-and-Education/Medicare-Learning-Network-MLN/MLNProducts/downloads/MedcrePhysFeeSchedfctsht.pdf

Work GPCI = Geographic Practice Cost Indices
PE = Practice Expense
MP = Malpractice Expense
CF = Conversion Factor

A dollar amount is assigned to the conversion factor and Medicare payments are calculated. Compensation from Medicare became RVU based in 1992 and, subsequently, most insurers have adopted similar compensation models. In December of 2013, several initiatives in the US Congress are attempting to modify the current payment system and incentivize both quality and integrated care.

One of the difficulties in medical practice results from insurance contracts. Virtually all insurance companies have slightly different fee schedules and mechanisms for billing. As a result, it is difficult to be certain that a given company is properly compensating a physician for a CPT code. Sophisticated computer systems and methods of checks and balances are required to assess the appropriateness of receipts.

Physicians must negotiate (or attempt to negotiate) compensation structures with each insurance carrier. Obviously, larger physician groups have more "clout" and the ability to receive better compensation; however, insurance companies do not have to negotiate if they have a high enough percentage of a given market; a physician might be unable to survive economically in such a circumstance if he did not agree with the insurer's terms. Of note, the Federal Trade Commission is interested in the consumer, not the provider, so it is unlikely to come to the assistance of physicians dealing with an insurance monopoly if the public is not harmed. Physicians who are not financially related (sharing risk) are not able to negotiate together with insurance companies. An attempt to do so would be considered collusion and a violation of federal law. Organizations of non-partner physicians such as IPAs (Independent Physician Associations) have limited ability to negotiate with insurers and must demonstrate quality improvement if they attempt to do so.

Traditional health insurance, which paid physicians based upon fee for service, has virtually disappeared in the United States and given way to managed care. There are two major forms of managed care: PPOs and HMOs. PPOs (preferred provider organizations) are insurance products that combine physicians, hospitals and other providers to provide care at a discounted rate. Typically, PPOs pay physicians based upon "discounted fee for service," which simply discounts the usual fee by a percentage or pays the physician a multiple of Medicare compensation. Most PPOs pay physicians an amount greater than Medicare. From the patient standpoint, PPOs place modest limits on physician and hospital choice. HMOs (health maintenance organizations) are insurance entities that typically have a "gatekeeper" primary care physician and drastically limit patient choice of physicians and hospitals. HMOs typically compensate physicians by either discounted fee for service or capitation. Capitation pays physicians a set sum to provide care for a group of patients for a given period of time. The physician is thus incentivized to limit care to only the necessary interactions.

Most leaders in health care economics believe that the fee for service system provides adverse incentives to physicians. This is not a new idea. The British literary giant George Bernard Shaw long ago grasped the dubious effects of fee-for-service medicine: In the preface to his 1909 play *The Doctor's Dilemma*, he lamented the payment norm that gave "a surgeon a pecuniary interest in cutting off your leg . . . and the more appalling the mutilation, the more the mutilator is paid." (Susan Dentzer. *Payment Reform: Parlous, And Yet Still Promising.* doi:10.1377/hlthaff.2012.0882 Health Aff September 2012 vol. 31 no. 9 1918). Innovative payment methods are clearly coming in the immediate future. There seem to be two major new ideas: bundled payments and ACOs.

Bundled payment is a concept in which all of the providers for an episode of care are paid a single lump sum—in essence, bundling the payment together. It is then up to the providers—hospital, physician, home health, etc.—to determine how the money will be split up. One can only imagine how contentious such deliberations might be if the providers are not integrated into a single entity. In fact, "integrated health care" in which all providers function together in an efficient manner is a method of achieving the goals of health care reform. The second novel approach is the ACO or accountable care organization. The Patient Protection and Affordable Care Act of 2010 allows for the creation of ACOs. ACOs are integrated health entities that provide care for a minimum of 5,000 Medicare patients and ultimately will be at risk for the financial aspects of their care. An ACO in some ways is the evolution of the HMO and compensation will likely be some form of capitation in the future. ACOs in Texas are problematic as they must, by Texas law, have physicians on their board of directors but funding will ultimately likely come from hospitals as they are the only current providers with enough money to deal with the necessary infrastructure and accept risk. Regardless of future compensation methods, it is clear that physician compensation will decrease.

Health Care Industry— The Medical Industrial Complex

Health care in the United States is "big money;" in fact, it is about 18% of the GDP. That number places the United States at the top of the developed world in terms of spending on health care. This is a bit misleading, as the 18% number includes medical device manufacturers, the pharmaceutical industry, and research. In fact, the United States spends more on health research than any other country. Nevertheless, the amount spent on health care is unsustainable. The graphs below demonstrate US spending vs. other countries. Note that the United States spends more money per capita and a higher percentage of the GDP than than any other country in the developed world. Although the United States spends enormous amounts of money on health care, the overall US population is less healthy than that of European countries. This is likely a result of poor access to care for a significant portion of our population; however, US survival is greater than that of European populations for complicated, technology-dependent illnesses. In addition, in the United States there is a negative correlation between Medicare spending and quality metrics.

Figure 13-4.

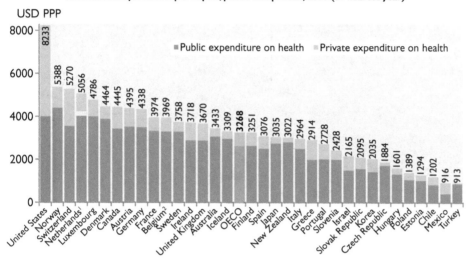

US spends two-and-a-half times the OECD average

Total health expenditure per capita, public and private, 2010 (or nearest year)

■ Public expenditure on health   ■ Private expenditure on health

1. In the Netherlands, it is not possible to clearly distinguish the public and private share related to investments.
2. Total expenditure excluding investments.
Information on data for Israel: http://dx.doi.org/10.1787/888932315602.

OECD Health Data 2012, *U.S. health care system from an international perspective*, Released on June 28, 2012
http://www.oecd.org/unitedstates/HealthSpendingInUSA_HealthData2012.pdf

Figure 13-5.

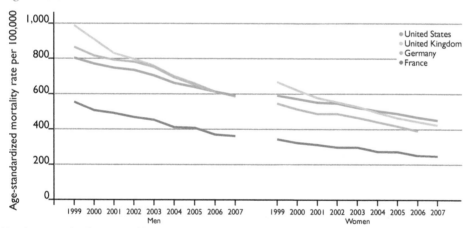

Trends in Mortality from Amenable Causes in Four Countries for People Ages 65–74, 1999–2006/2007.
"SOURCE: Authors' calculations based on data from the World Health Organization mortality database
(Note 15 in text) and Centers for Disease Control and Prevention vital statistics data (Note 16 in text).
NOTE: Data for Germany for 2007 were not available." *Health Affairs* 31, no. 9 (September 2012): 2114–2122.

Exhibit 13-6. International Comparison of Spending on Health, 1980-2007

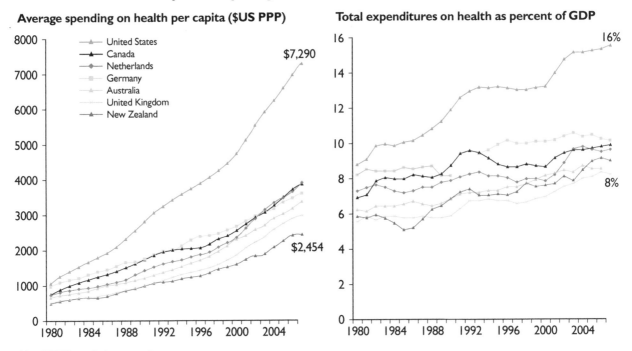

Average spending on health per capita ($US PPP)

- United States
- Canada
- Netherlands
- Germany
- Australia
- United Kingdom
- New Zealand

$7,290

$2,454

Total expenditures on health as percent of GDP

16%

8%

Note: $US PPP = purchasing power parity.

Source: Organization for Economic Cooperation and Development, *OECD Health Data, 2009* (Paris: OECD, Nov. 2009).

Source: Centers for Medicare & Medicaid Services, Office of the Actuary, National Health Statistics Group.

From *Mirror, Mirror on the Wall: How the Performance of the U.S. Health Care System Compares Internationally, 2010 Update* by The Commonwealth Fund. Copyright © 2010 by The Commonwealth Fund. Reprinted by permission.

As is evident from the preceding graphs, health care spending in the United States is enormous. Much of this spending is the over-reliance on technology that occurs in our country. The influence of the pharmaceutical industry and medical device manufacturers is obvious to anyone who watches prime time television. The ACA currently has significant taxes for both of these industries although this is likely to change.

Both the pharmaceutical industry and medical device manufacturers currently subtly influence physician behavior by paying physicians to perform "research" on their products or to speak at conferences about diseases amenable to treatment by their products. The ACA has sunshine provisions that will hopefully render such arrangements transparent to consumers. Nevertheless, physicians must have the moral insight to determine conflicts of interest when they exist and be certain that their patients receive optimal care.

Physician compensation accounts for about 20–30% of the health care dollar; however, physician behavior is the driving force behind the majority of health care spending. Current and future medical education will clearly address the issues of efficiency in the system and the push to have an integrated delivery system will necessarily gain momentum. The era of fee for service medicine provided by doctors in solo or small practices is coming to an end.

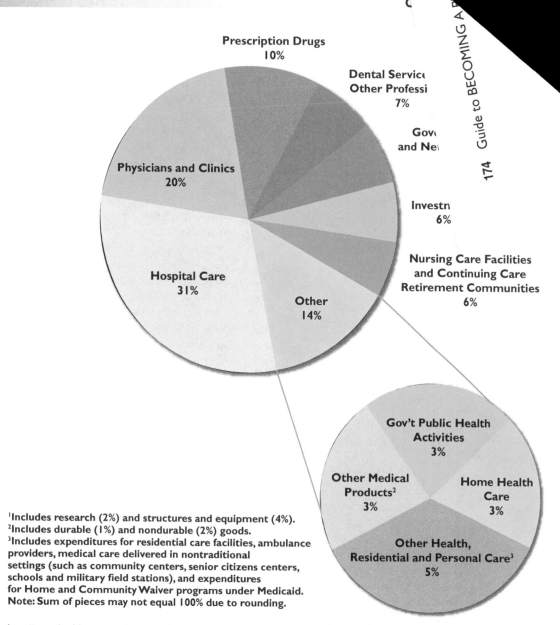

Prescription Drugs
10%

Dental Service
Other Professi
7%

Gov
and Ne

Investn
6%

Physicians and Clinics
20%

Hospital Care
31%

Other
14%

Nursing Care Facilities
and Continuing Care
Retirement Communities
6%

Gov't Public Health
Activities
3%

Other Medical
Products²
3%

Home Health
Care
3%

Other Health,
Residential and Personal Care³
5%

¹Includes research (2%) and structures and equipment (4%).
²Includes durable (1%) and nondurable (2%) goods.
³Includes expenditures for residential care facilities, ambulance
providers, medical care delivered in nontraditional
settings (such as community centers, senior citizens centers,
schools and military field stations), and expenditures
for Home and Community Waiver programs under Medicaid.
Note: Sum of pieces may not equal 100% due to rounding.

http://www.healthcareandreform.com/locations/washington/individuals-and-families/the-reform-challenge
/where-your-dollar-goes/

Reflections of a Hospital Administrator

By William Neilson, MS, MD

Courtesy John W. Neilson

As a Chief Medical Officer who practiced in academia, a large group, a small group, and ultimately an employed arrangement, I have a unique perspective on hospital-physician relationships. Hospitals and physicians typically have a rocky relationship, primarily because their incentives are different. Under today's system, physicians are rewarded for performing more procedures, seeing more patients, and keeping patients in the hospital longer. There are relatively trivial amounts of money tied to quality metrics for physicians. In contrast, hospitals are incentivized to move patients through the system rapidly, discharge patients at the earliest possible moment, and meet very complex quality metrics to maintain or improve payment rates. Furthermore, meeting hospital quality metrics is almost totally dependent upon physician behavior, yet physicians have virtually no incentive to follow the metrics.

As a result of the opposing incentives, hospitals feel forced to try to create integrated systems with employed (or at least contracted) physicians. This, of course, creates intense angst amongst those physicians who are not employed and are not sympathetic with the hospitals' attempts to meet quality metrics and improve efficiency.

Hospital administrators have invariably been trained to understand Six Sigma, a manufacturing concept that improves efficiency and minimizes variation. One can only imagine how frustrated hospital administrators are when each hip replacement patient receives totally different orders in a different sequence by each orthopedist. The likelihood of error and poor results is greatly magnified and the medical staff is oblivious. The obvious reason is that physicians have no training in process improvement and some even believe that reducing variation creates "cookbook" medicine which, in their minds, creates poor care.

Further increasing the divide between physicians and hospitals is competition. In the somewhat distant past, most ancillary services (lab, x-ray, etc.) were provided in the hospital and were (and still are) major profit centers for hospitals. As technology has improved and become cheaper, more and more physicians provide the ancillary services that were once reserved for the hospital. As a result, hospital bottom lines have suffered and physician incomes have increased or at least stabilized. Hospitals can do little to avert this problem, as it is illegal to incentivize physicians to use hospital services. This is yet another impetus for hospitals to employ physicians. Furthermore, especially in Texas, there was a move to create new physician-owned specialty hospitals. Such hospitals typically provide highly profitable outpatient or short stay surgical procedures such as might be provided by an otolaryngologist or orthopedist. These facilities do not provide significant care for the indigent; in fact, many surgeons will take their indigent patients to the community hospital and their paying patients to their specialty hospital. Creation of such a hospital in my community removed ~$15,000,000 from the bottom line of the non-profit community hospital. Obviously, the financial incentive for the surgeon to participate in hospital profits through an ownership interest is huge, and it is illegal for a hospital to compete with such a development by incentivizing physicians not to participate. The ACA placed a moratorium on building new physician-owned hospitals or expanding existing hospitals and fixed the percent of ownership by physicians at the March 2010 level. Of course, physician-owned hospitals can opt out of Medicare and not be subject to the rules of the ACA.

Perhaps the most frustrating issue of all involves the responsibility that hospitals have to ensure quality care within their walls. The ultimate responsibility for quality care resides with the hospital board of trustees, but they delegate this to the organized medical staff. The conflict comes from the inability of hospitals to assess quality;

only a physician can typically determine whether or not appropriate care has been provided to a patient. Hospitals must find physicians who are willing to volunteer their time to evaluate (and perhaps discipline) their peers—a task that is thankless and potentially risky. What cardiac surgeon is going to criticize the care of his referring cardiologist? I personally was threatened with a $1,000,000+ lawsuit for revoking a fellow surgeon's privileges when I was president of my hospital's medical staff. Hospital administrators need the help of the medical staff to create protocols, lead departments, and serve on committees. Such work is frequently voluntary and, if paid, subject to Stark law provisions. The administrator must find a way to inspire the medical staff to take responsibility and improve quality.

The practice of medicine is a great joy, but the business of medicine is frequently unpleasant. Its complexity is frustrating to doctors who simply want to care for the sick. The management guru Peter Drucker once said, "Even small health care institutions are complex, barely manageable places . . . Large health care institutions may be the most complex organizations in human history." This must surely be true.

© Kendall Hunt Publishing Company

Money and Medicine Reflection

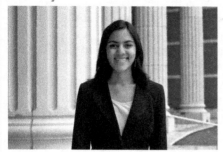

By Shreya Goyal
Baylor College of Medicine, Class of 2019

When pursuing a career in healthcare, you may hear phrases such as "medicine is changing, you know" or "medicine is not what it used to be in the past." These phrases typically refer to the recent changes brought about through legislation such as the Affordable Care Act (ACA) and new compensation structures for physicians. As a former business major and a current medical student, I am aware that it is very important to understand the financial implications of pursuing a career in medicine; the large price tag that comes with becoming a doctor is yet another reason it is essential to ensure that you truly want to become a physician.

In order to become a physician, there are a few financial considerations to keep in mind. Be ready to not earn a penny until residency. Not only will you be forgoing potential income, but you may also be amassing a large amount of debt: medical school is expensive no matter where you choose to go. While new physicians graduate with high earning potential, they also have 4–8 years of debt from pursuing a medical education. However, there are several options to finance your medical education along the way or reduce your debt. When choosing a medical school, it is important to note that public medical schools are cheaper on average than private medical schools. In order to offset the debt you incur from your undergraduate to resident years, you can apply for scholarships. Scholarships exist for virtually every level of experience, starting from your high school years to your fourth year of medical school. These applications are highly competitive, of course, so be sure to apply early!

The federal government also offers various programs to refinance your student loans. These programs are targeted at medical residents who will work in Health Professional Shortage Areas (HPSAs) for 3 years after graduating from medical school. The government provides the residents with tuition and stipend reimbursements for each year of service in an HPSA. Additionally, due to a shortage of primary care physicians in the United States, the National Health Service Corps has created healthcare loan repayment programs in which primary care residents commit to working at least 2 of 3 years in an underserved area of the United States for loan repayment of up to $120,000. Alternatively, you can also opt to apply for an MD/PhD program or work in the military, both of which may pay for your medical school tuition.

continued

Money and Medicine Reflection *(continued)*

Another financial aspect to consider is the specialty you would like to pursue. Of course, each specialty comes with its own positives and drawbacks. The biggest financial incentive of pursuing a highly competitive field (e.g., neurosurgery or dermatology) for some is the high income associated with the specialty; however, note that the more specialized the field, the more years of training and education you will need before you can practice, which could potentially lead to more years of unpaid debt. Also, depending on which specialty you choose, malpractice insurance premiums vary vastly based upon the complexity of services and associated risks and complications.

Furthermore, once you have completed your training, you will need to decide whether you want to work in a hospital-setting, group practice, or solo practice. As mentioned in this chapter, there are several advantages and disadvantages to each of these. Depending on which work setting you are a part of will determine how you get paid and the benefits you receive. For example, while working in a hospital and serving patients through Accountable Care Organizations (ACOs), a physician will have to share profits and risks with the hospital and other providers; meanwhile, in a private practice, a new physician may have to pay to enter the practice, not participate in a strong retirement plan, or not have the opportunity to work with the latest, most innovative medical equipment and technology. With the new ACA legislation, the healthcare industry is transforming from a volume-based approach to value-based approach. As a consequence of shifting from focusing on quantity of care to quality of care, medical professionals are now being reimbursed based on improvement in patient outcomes rather than the number of procedures and services provided.

If you find medical school tuition figures daunting, these are all key considerations to becoming debt-free in a shorter amount of time compared to most graduates. Through these measures, when you become the medical doctor you have always dreamed of becoming, you can actually enjoy the fruits of your labor instead of worrying about repaying your student loans.

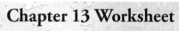

Chapter 13 Worksheet

Have you thought about your future income
and medical practice?

Make a list of the most challenging issues you will have managing your medical career and medical practice in regards to the financial and legal challenges that impact the health professions.

1)

2)

3)

4)

5)

6)

7)

What is your plan to manage the debt from your medical school and undergraduate education?

What type of medical setting (hospital, private practice, medical school) do you wish to practice medicine in? What are the financial or practical benefits and challenges of this particular setting?

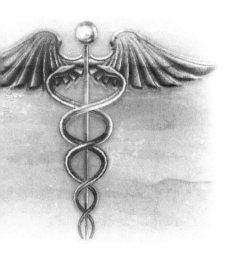

Chapter 14
Family and Medicine

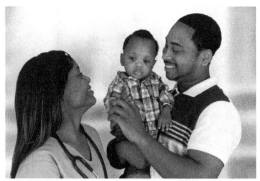

© Rob Mamion, 2014. Used under license from Shutterstock, Inc.

Work-life balance is important and has been a hot topic for a long time especially in the realm of medicine. This balance has come to the forefront as more and more households are double income, meaning both partners work. Recently, there has been some debate in the media and self-help reading about whether men and women can "have it all." The question is: Can a career man or woman have a successful and demanding career and balance a successful and demanding home life? There are many opinions on this. Some say it is possible, while others say that it is not realistic. No matter how you feel, it is important to take into account what you want in the future as you choose your career.

Although medicine is changing as our culture changes, it continues to be a self-sacrificing profession. Physicians will put their patients first, which means family may take a second seat at times. If a devoted physician has a patient crashing during family dinnertime, dinner will be missed. If the hospital needs coverage during the holidays, a holiday may be missed. These types of needs and emergencies will vary among medical professions, but the common denominator is the devotion physicians feel for their craft.

In order to have a full picture of what to expect regarding a career in medicine and family, some physicians and a medical student have shared their work-life balance: the good, the bad, and the ugly; how they have coped with the challenges of balancing their career with their personal life; and what they do and do not recommend.

Drs. Jim & Rhonda Walton

It's safe to say that balancing the lives of two actively practicing physicians and a house full of children is enough to bring anyone to their knees. It is true that the challenge of finding and then maintaining balance is an elusive goal. We have achieved periods of work-life balance, but maintaining a sense of accomplishment in this area stressed our type-A personalities to the breaking point more than once. As physicians, we had

continued

Drs. Jim & Rhonda Walton *(continued)*

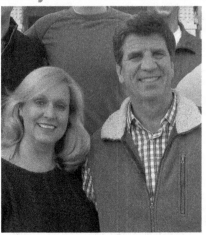

grown accustomed to mastering the things we diligently attempted, but we quickly learned that the academic disciplines of medical school were significantly different than the disciplines required for family life management.

One of the most important pieces of advice we ever received was that we needed to realize and accept we would fail many times in maintaining a sense of mastery over our family life, sometimes miserably, but success would be defined by "continuing to show up." At the time, this seemed like relatively simplistic advice. However, over time, we came to appreciate its wisdom. Much like medical school, it seemed that "showing up" would be more difficult than we thought, particularly during times of discouragement, disappointment, and interpersonal stress. However, the rule held true that as we stubbornly refused to lose ourselves in the busyness of our practices, we were often rewarded with surprises of success in our private lives. Physicians learn much of what they know about medicine through the use of case studies. Typically, inside a case study there are nuggets of challenging diagnostic or therapeutic lessons that forever cement the much sought-after knowledge. It is in the case study where physicians learn to "never forget" the mistake or lesson learned, sometimes in a very painful and stubborn reminder of our fallibility (and occasionally brilliance). The stories below are a few of our "case studies" in family balance.

Jim: When Rhonda was a first-year resident, only four months after delivering our first son, I practiced in a local urgent care clinic doing shift work to pay back some of our student loans. We were working diligently to reduce our medical education debt so we alternated our residency training. Rhonda started her pediatric residency and I planned to do internal medicine after she was done. Back then you could work as a general practitioner in urgent care clinics with only one year of residency training. Our first son, Steven, was only a few months old and I became his primary care giver while Rhonda worked the long hours of a resident. Every third night she spent the night taking care of new admissions and critically ill children in the NICU of the Children's hospital. It became a ritual for me to meet Rhonda for dinner with our baby son, spending most of the evening waiting for her to have a break between her patient care to spend time together. I got to know many of her colleagues over those long hours, and Steven got to spend time with his mom, albeit in a non-traditional way.

During those years when Rhonda wasn't working the night shift, she was home late in the evening, exhausted with only a few hours to spend any family time before fatigue overwhelmed her and sleep became a necessity. One of the lessons I learned here was that my traditional view of masculinity would need some adjustment if I wanted to be a successful father. I was blessed to have a healthy son, who would grow to enjoy sharing with his dad the many fun and exciting things of boyhood, but in this early stage, he needed time with his busy and overworked mother. Three years of this pattern set into motion a balancing act around time management that continues to this day.

Rhonda: I can't say I would necessarily recommend having a baby at the end of medical school right before starting a residency, but managing a 90-hour work week as a new mom did provide opportunities for "creative thinking." It also reinforced the importance of partnering with someone who understands and embraces your passion before attempting to pursue a career in medicine and having a family. Training in pediatrics made me fairly confident in the specifics of mothering, but delegating the primary childcare responsibilities to my husband proved unnerving. When I bathed the baby, I carefully checked the water temperature, swaddled him in a warm towel, and gently cleansed his eyelids with a moist cotton ball, only to come home the next day to find Jim standing naked in the shower holding our screaming, slippery newborn up under the shower head. My career gave me countless such opportunities to discover that my spouse was a caring, competent parent even though he didn't do everything exactly as I would have. Knowing that Jim would bring our son to the hospital and patiently wait for me to have an unpredictable break when we could be together made it bearable to spend so many hours taking care of other people's kids.

The lifelong journey of dealing with "working-mom" guilt began when I gave birth and continues today as I watch my adult children make adult decisions. I remember attending a women's Bible study on a rare evening off. A woman I had just met publically berated me for working full time. She explained that God calls women to be wives and mothers and that if I really loved my children and called myself a Christian, I would give up my selfish rebellion and devote myself to raising my children and supporting my husband's career. I tearfully thought back to my college years when I had felt so strongly that God was calling me to serve Him as a physician, and I wondered if I had been confused. Only a few days later, the very same woman called me at 2:00 a.m. asking advice about her sick child and speaking as if we were best friends. I patiently advised her, not needing to point out that she couldn't have it both ways, because I gratefully realized that she had given me a great gift. God is capable of complexity and He expects us to be as well. There are no preset roles for women (or men, or couples); we are individually called to do specific and sometimes difficult things based on our giftedness, not our gender. We are to work out the "division of labor" in a marriage based on what works, not on some culturally mandated hierarchy, and when God calls us to serve Him, He doesn't forget we have kids.

Jim: After Rhonda finished her residency and during the second year of my internal medicine residency, Rhonda delivered our second son, Daniel. She had just started her private practice, partnering with another established physician in a small community practice. Both of our work hours were long and we were fortunate to have a babysitter that could care for Steven at our home. Rhonda's schedule was more flexible and she now had a day off during the week. However, after-hours and weekend phone calls were frequent and disruptions in family time were common.

My residency hours were predictably long and limited my energy and time for participation in caring for Steven (and Rhonda). Nevertheless, it was important to us that we space our children so that they were no more than three years apart. We were excited to be having another son and Rhonda's pregnancy went as well as it could, since most of it was during her third year of her Pediatric residency. I think she showed super-human strength during the second pregnancy, balancing her resident work obligations, and caring for Steven while I was a first-year resident.

What we didn't expect or plan for was a sick baby. Daniel was born at term, but he had a rare condition called persistent fetal circulation. The condition left him on a mechanical ventilator in the NICU for a month and once his survival was assured, we took him home on an infant monitor that seemed to beep incessantly throughout the night. For months, Daniel struggled to recover from his difficult start.

We learned over these months that our rather simplistic, well-planned formula for adding children and creating a family along with two medical careers could lead to unplanned disruptions. Our career trajectories were forever altered by the birth of our second son. We were startled to learn that we were vulnerable and unable to "control" our lives as easily as we thought we could. Within a matter of 90 short days, we found ourselves deciding to move closer to family for much needed emotional and physical support to help our small family thrive while maintaining our career commitments. This decision created a need for both Rhonda and me to disconnect from our respective medical communities where we worked. As a result, we left the medium-sized city of Dayton, Ohio, where we were living and working, and I transferred to another internal medicine residency program in Dallas while Rhonda opened a solo practice in a small town south of Dallas Fort Worth closer to her parents.

continued

Drs. Jim & Rhonda Walton *(continued)*

Rhonda: Those who end up in medical school are often "planners" by nature. This is a trait that serves us well. The rigors of a medical education and then the demands of a busy practice require planning, organization, and superior time-management skills. Family life; however, requires flexibility and resilience, especially when carefully constructed plans go terribly wrong.

Having a baby fighting for his life in the NICU was never in my plan, but that painful experience taught us both a great deal about supporting each other and about receiving support from others.

Practicing medicine allows a privileged entry into the most intimate, emotional, and vulnerable spaces of our patients' lives. As physicians, our own complicated, unexpected family stressors often become valuable resources to draw on when walking through those experiences with patients.

For me, this "relational" part of a primary care practice has provided the most precious rewards (and the most annoying interruptions) of being a pediatrician. I've known the difficulty of keeping my emotions in check while taking care of a critically ill child with meningitis who happened to be the same age as one of my own children. I've had great fun sitting on a bleacher at my son's baseball game when a sweet patient, waving the asthma inhaler I gave him, ran up and flashed a toothless grin, gave me a hug, and said, "Look, Doctor Walton, I can be on the team now!" It was less fun when enjoying a rare romantic dinner with my husband and someone I wasn't sure I recognized interrupted us with, "Hey, Doc, Jacob hasn't pooped in a week. What should we do?" I sometimes found myself buying groceries at 1:00 a.m. because I was less likely to run into patients wanting medical advise in the produce section of HEB.

Practicing general pediatrics in a small Texas town provided the family and community support we needed as we raised our four young sons, but the balancing act was no less difficult. Since I covered pediatric backup for the delivery room, the nursery, and the ER, the beeper was a constant reminder to my children that I might be called away at any moment in the middle of any activity. I missed some milestones and field trips and ball games, but I showed up for most of them, usually at the expense of getting the amount of sleep considered healthy for humans.

Jim's call schedule was even more demanding than mine when we were both in private practice, and it seemed most days that the primary responsibilities of child care fell on my shoulders. We took turns attending kids' activities in the evenings, but when one of them woke up with a fever, it was up to me to make sure I had backup arrangements. The maternal guilt raised its head on a regular basis. But looking back, I don't remember any of the kids ever expressing resentment about either of us being called away to take care of patients. In fact, the boys would sometimes bring random friends with medical complaints to our house for us to take care of. I like to think that our choices set an example of being "others centered" and gave them opportunities to develop resilience and flexibility.

Jim: Over the last decade, we have seen the medical profession evolve to accommodate the challenges of work-life balance, understanding that the new generation of physicians (both men and women) were going to demand more appreciation and respect for their personal lives. This has led to more flexibility in the type of work hours and created more opportunities for the practice of medicine to approximate the "typical 8–5 job" as opposed to traditional "unlimited time" for the professional calling. Nevertheless, these accommodations that enable physicians to better control their patients' access must be seen essentially dependent upon where you choose to live and work or your specialty. For example, if you choose to practice medicine in a rural setting, you may not have the same level of collegial support as you would if you practiced in a suburban or urban setting. Additionally, depending upon your specialty training, you may find yourself as the only specialist of your kind for miles around (with an unlimited demand for your time and talent). On the other hand, you may be one of literally hundreds of specialists within an urban setting struggling to keep your practice full. In short, there is no panacea or short-cut method to creating the skills necessary to balance family and work (no matter what profession or job).

Rhonda: The challenges of work-life balance eventually led to the decision to add multiple part-time pediatric partners. This creative solution helped address many of the time pressures we experienced and also helped establish a new culture for our practice. I was able to have a job-sharing situation where I had more time off during the week and could spend more time with the children after school. Later, I left private practice to work in an inner city charity clinic in Dallas. The pediatricians in the group I started over 20 years ago now have an exclusively outpatient practice. There are hospitalists to cover inpatient calls, so the dreaded nighttime trek to the hospital is rare for general pediatricians. Primary care medicine seems to have evolved some over the years to be a bit more "family friendly," at least in some practices. But as I visit with young physicians, especially female physicians, I find that the external pressure (from family, friends, church, etc. . . .) to fulfill some preconceived gender role in family life seems to still be pervasive. It is clear to me that, for most physicians, finding the strength to be confident in the unique, unscripted ways they make their own family work is as challenging as surviving sleepless nights or making difficult diagnoses.

© Kendall Hunt Publishing Company

Reflections

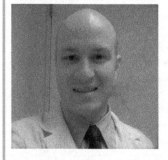

By Jason R. Jones, MD, MS
Texas A&M Health Science Center College of
*   Medicine, 2014*
University of North Texas Health Science Center, MS
*   in Medical Science, 2010*
Southwestern University, BS, Biology, 2007

For most of my undergraduate years, I was a single guy who imagined that a spouse and family would be a characteristic of my life, well after medical school. It just made sense to do all that hard work for my family and not put them through it. Honestly, I probably wasn't mature enough at that time to think or plan the activities of the next day, much less aspects of my life that required a high level of commitment such as medical school or a family. I question my maturity by citing the evidence of a foolishly underdeveloped pre-med experience and an application as strong as a spaghetti noodle. You'd think that if I were not ready to start my medical education that I'd have no business getting married. Let me tell you, you're probably right! But as I look back on the decade since meeting my wife, I recognize that I wouldn't be making my residency rank list for a very competitive specialty, full of many prestigious institutions, without my wife and baby girl.

We are creatures of habit that seek comfort within familiarity. As you've probably heard, medical school and a physician's career will take however much time you give it. Should you want to spend a hundred and twenty hours a week with work and study, the profession will gladly accept that from you. If you want to skip class and study just an hour on weekdays, it will take that much too. Now you're quick enough to know that somewhere in-between is a healthy and prudent level of commitment for success, but discovering what is right for you is a rather difficult task. We all seek familiarity in patterns of work that still afford time for our brains to unwind, not unlike a child who thrives within a school's structure but is given time to play and be free. In other words, organized study habits and a solid work ethic must be "balanced" with time spent free of the stressors of our daily lives. Not exclusive to the medical field, folks find their retreat in exercise, reading, television, movies, *Breaking Bad*, and cooking, just to name a few. For me, my retreat is family.

I love that my family needs me like I need them. They will notice if I spend all weekend at the library or pull an all-nighter. They will know if I am stressing about the

continued

Reflections *(continued)*

upcoming STEP exam that I have been avoiding. They will notice the empty seat at the dinner table if I stay up late at the anatomy lab. They will know when my choices cost them time with their husband or father. I love that my enjoyment for this time with my family causes me to be exceedingly efficient and entirely committed to utilizing the workday hours to their fullest. I feel that it is unrealistic to expect to reach your potential in medical school in a forty-hour workweek, but it is not impractical to concentrate your efforts around that same workweek with some additional effort applied at other times. For example, many Friday and Saturday nights were spent in the school library, shoulder to shoulder with my wife. She worked on lesson plans for her school as I studied and learned. Sharing that time seemed to create a sense of mutual investment in each other's career. By spending this time as a couple on our work, Sundays could be enjoyed together without stress or worry. I wonder how "balanced" my life would be without my wife and baby girl. It's safe to say that Walter White wouldn't care if I skipped an episode or two to spend more time at school.

There are unavoidable times in this field that truly test a family. During many clinical rotations, you are out of the house well before dawn and back around supper, six days a week. Some folks in residency entertain that schedule for five or more years! There are frequent nights spent entirely at the hospital, listening to pagers unceasingly sing their love songs. It's taxing, no matter how you look at it: as a couple, family, or single. One can't help but be jealous at times of the single classmates who have no one missing them at home while they wait for that surgeon to make up their mind or for that baby to hurry up and join their birthday party. But with ever-renewed patience for me by my family—and for my family by me—we are making it and enjoying it!

I'll conclude with an anecdote about this career path and having a family. I have had the pleasure of serving on the Admissions Committee for our College of Medicine. One of my favorite things about the role is reading and hearing the various reasons why applicants come to this field. I am energized by their stories and their lives. In their unique experiences, I identify, remember, and discover new reasons for committing to this vocation. Medical students will inevitably reach a point when they question why they are there. For some, it may be after they get their first exam grade, and for others it may be on one of those nights when the pager song has awoken them for the fifth time. It's an overwhelming feeling of fear and doubt, seeming to articulate that no paycheck can make this feeling right. You see, somewhere along the way, with all the stress we put on ourselves as med students, we lose our reason for being here and we question everything. When some feel all alone there, I tap the home button on my iPhone and see my beautiful, loving, and supportive wife gaze with admiration upon our daughter who is eating Fig Newtons in the bed and leaving crumbs for Daddy. That undergraduate vision of finding my wife after it was all said and done wasn't meant to be. Fortuitously, the story written in its place has been far sweeter and I will be a much better physician because of it.

Conclusions

Medicine is a demanding but rewarding profession. There are many types of medical specialties that have unique lifestyle options that can be considered. Clearly, a career in medicine will present some challenges in balancing personal interests and family responsibilities, but it certainly can be managed. Nevertheless, premedical students need to thoughtfully consider their personal values and decide whether or not the opportunities provided by a career in medicine are worth some of the personal sacrifices. As with any career, it is important to discover the appropriate fit for one's personal goals and lifestyle.

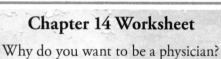

Chapter 14 Worksheet

Why do you want to be a physician?

Reflect back through the work you have completed throughout this course and what you have learned about a career in medicine. Similar to the exercise in Chapter 1, write your reasons for wanting to be a physician at this point.

1)

2)

3)

4)

5)

6)

7)

What was added? What was subtracted from the previous list? What is the biggest change?

How do you plan on balancing a family life with your medical career? What issues to feel you will have to face or work through to be a both a successful parent and physician?

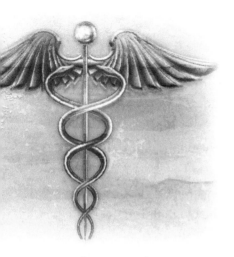

Key Terms

Academic Fresh Start: Program in Texas allowing coursework 10 years old and older to be ignored for enrollment purposes and from being calculated into the GPA.

Alternate List/Waitlist: List of applicants a medical school has interviewed that have yet to receive an offer of admission.

American Association of Colleges of Osteopathic Medicine Application Service (AACOMAS): Central application service for all DO programs in the United States, except the DO medical school in Texas which uses TMDSAS. https://aacomas.aacom.org/

Accreditation Council for Graduate Medical Education (ACGME): This organization is responsible for accrediting residency and fellowship education programs.

American Medical Association (AMA): This organization is designed to promote and propel the field of medicine. It serves both social and political purposes as well as offering services to the physician community.

American Medical College Application Service (AMCAS): Central application service for all MD programs in the United States (including Puerto Rico), except the Texas public medical schools, which use TMDSAS. https://www.aamc.org/students/applying/amcas/

Association of American Medical Colleges (AAMC): The nonprofit association representing all accredited US and 17 Canadian MD granting programs as well as teaching hospitals and health systems, and Department of Veterans Affairs. https://www.aamc.org/

American Association of Colleges Of Osteopathic Medicine (AACOM): The nonprofit association representing the 31 accredited colleges of osteopathic medicine in the United States. http://www.aacom.org

American Osteopathic Association (AOA): This organization serves as the primary certifying body for Osteopathic physicians.

Attending Physician: In an educational institution, there are teams of medical students, residents, and fellows. The board certified physician leading the team is often referred to as an attending physician.

Behavioral Interview Questions: These questions are often used in interviews as they have shown to have better predictive value for an applicant's behavior. The questions are situational and focus on past experiences and behaviors.

BCPM GPA: Biology, Chemistry, Physics, and Mathematics Grade Point Average. Medical schools will isolate the specific grades from these academic areas to evaluate applicants.

Blind Interview: An interview format that provides very little information to the interviewer about the applicant.

Closed-File Interview: An interview format that provides very little data to the interviewer about the applicant. This may include biographical data and no academic information.

Comprehensive Osteopathic Medical Licensing Examination (COMLEX): Licensing exam for DO medical students.

Curriculum Viate (CV): This document serves as a listing of education, professional experience, awards, publications and any other accomplishments that may relate to a career. This document will change and grow throughout a person's career.

Dean's Letter: Also known as the MSPE, this letter is a summary of medical student performance throughout all 4 years of their UGME career.

Doctor of Medicine (MD): The degree earned in allopathic medicine.

Doctor of Osteopathic Medicine (DO): The degree earned in osteopathic medicine.

Electronic Residency Application Service (ERAS): Central application service for GME, which includes most ACGME accredited programs.

Family Education Rights and Privacy Act (FERPA): A Federal law that protects the privacy of student education records. http://www2.ed.gov/policy/gen/guid/fpco/ferpa/index.html

Fellowship: Traditionally a period of sub-specialty training that follows residency or another fellowship.

Fee Assistance Program (FAP): Program through AAMC that provides those with financial need a reduced cost to take the MCAT. https://www.aamc.org/students/applying/fap/

Grade Point Average (GPA): The average of all course grades taken in college and graduate school.

Graduate Medical Education (GME): This term is used to describe medical training following medical school graduation. Both residency and fellowship fall under the umbrella of GME.

Health Insurance Portability and Accountability ACT (HIPPA): A federal law (1996) designed to make it easier for patients to keep health insurance, protect the confidentiality and security of healthcare information and help the healthcare industry control administrative cost. If you are interested in shadowing or volunteering in a clinical setting, you will need to have certified training of HIPPA. http://www.hhs.gov/ocr/privacy/

Holistic Admissions: The approach some medical schools to look all aspects of an applicant's file to make decisions, rather than just relying on metrics.

The AAMC has developed a formal program called Holistic Review Project: https://www.aamc.org/initiatives/holisticreview/

Internship: The first year of a medical residency program is traditionally classified as internship.

Joint Degrees (Dual Degrees): Programs allowing a student to earn an additional degree to the MD/DO.

Medical College Admission Test (MCAT): The exam required for entry into medical school. https://www.aamc.org/students/applying/mcat/

Medical School Admissions Requirements (MSAR): A guide published by the AAMC with matriculation data, requirements for admissions, and financing. https://www.aamc.org/students/applying/requirements/msar/

Medical School Match: Process used by the TMDSAS schools to fill seats in each of the school's classes and occurs at the beginning of February.

Medical Student Performance Evaluation (MSPE): Formerly known as the Dean's Letter.

Multiple Mini-Interview (MMI): An interview format that uses several short independent assessments, typically in a timed circuit.

National Matching Services (NMS): Central application system for AOA GME programs.

Nontraditional Applicant: An applicant can be considered nontraditional by many factors including having a previous career, earning a graduate degree prior to applying, having served active duty in the military, or being 25 years old or older at the time of matriculation to medical school.

Open-File Interview: An interview format that may provide all the applicant's information to an interviewer.

Osteopathic Manipulative Medicine: Set of techniques DO students learn to attempt to diagnose and treat somatic dysfunction by manipulating a person's bones and muscles.

Pre-Match: Process used by the TMDSAS schools allowing schools to make offers between November 15th and December 31st.

PubMed: Online abstract database for health related peer-reviewed research articles http://www.ncbi.nlm.nih.gov/pubmed

Residency: A period of specialty training that follows medical school.

Rotations/Clerkships: Clinical rotations during the clinical years of medical school where students can gain exposure to various specialties of medicine.

Scribe: A paid position working in a hospital or clinic to chart notes for physicians as they see patients.

Secondary/Supplemental Application: The additional applications some medical schools required in addition to the primary application.

Shadowing: The act of volunteering to follow a physician (or other professional) as they go about their work in order to gain exposure to the field.

Texas Medical and Dental Schools Application Service (TMDSAS): Central application service for Texas public medical schools. https://www.tmdsas. com/

Undergraduate Medical Education (UGME): Medical school is classified as undergraduate medical education.

United States Medical Licensing Examination (USMLE): Licensing exam for all MD students.